Workouts for Working People

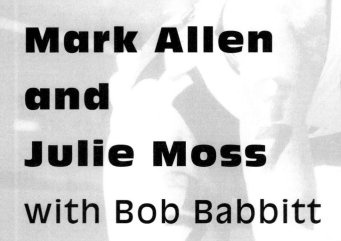

Mark Allen
and
Julie Moss

with Bob Babbitt

Villard Books 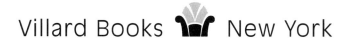 New York

Workouts for Working People

How You Can Get in
Great Shape While
Staying Employed

Copyright © 2000 by Mark Allen and Julie Moss

All rights reserved under International and Pan-American Copyright Conventions. Published in the United States by Villard Books, a division of Random House, Inc., New York, and simultaneously in Canada by Random House of Canada Limited, Toronto.

Photography credits:
Page 136 courtesy Bud Light USTS Series; pages 36, 144: Tracy Frankel; page 6: Carol Hogan; page 146: Diane Johnson; pages 64–82: Tim Mantoani; page 17: Mike Plant; pages 4, 5, 10, 22, 26, 29, 32, 33, 35, 43, 49, 55, 61, 118, 122, 127, 139, 149, 150: Lois Schwartz

VILLARD BOOKS is a registered trademark of Random House, Inc.

Library of Congress Cataloging-in-Publication Data

Allen, Mark, 1958–
Workouts for working people: how you can get in great shape while staying employed / Mark Allen and Julie Moss with Bob Babbitt.
p.   cm.
ISBN 0-375-75270-6 (alk. paper)
1. Physical fitness.   2. Exercise.   I. Moss, Julie.   II. Babbitt, Bob.   III. Title.
GV481.A43   2000
613.7—dc21   99-38824

Random House website address: www.atrandom.com

Printed in the United States of America on acid-free paper

2 3 4 5 6 7 8 9

First Edition

BOOK DESIGN BY JESSICA SHATAN

This book is dedicated

to PHIL MAFFETONE, for helping us discover the real art of training;

to DIANE BUCHTA, who shared with us her love of strength training and proved to us that endurance athletes can truly benefit from its use;

to MIKE RUBANO, whose knowledge of body movement led to our flexibility program; and

to BRANT SECUNDA, whose help made the impossible possible and without whom these stories would be very different.

And a special dedication to our son MATS, who loves being physical and likes nothing better than to go for a run through the neighborhood with Mom and Dad.

Acknowledgments

We would like to acknowledge some of the people who shared our vision for this book: Mollie Doyle and Scott Waxman for believing in us, nutritionist Nancy Ling for her expertise and patience, and copy editor Beth Hagman for her hard work and dedication. Special thanks go to our photographers—and friends—Lois Schwartz, Tracy Frankel, Rich Cruse, Tim Mantoani, and Tony Di Zinno. A book like this requires a team effort. And we were lucky enough to have the best team in the business.

Contents

Part I

Get Started

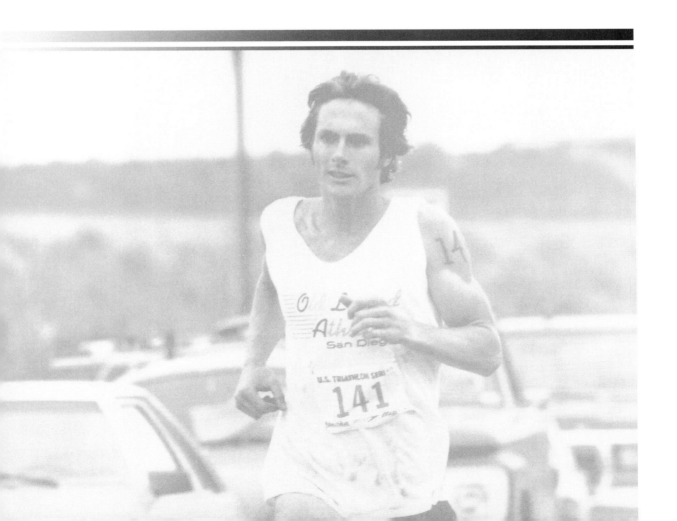

1 How We Began

The goal of life is to die young as late
as possible.

—Anthropologist Ashley Montagu

The call came from *Outside* magazine. It was one of those good news/bad news things. "Mark," said the voice on the other end, "we want to do a training article featuring you as the World's Fittest Man. We need to set up a date for a photo shoot as soon as possible."

Gulp.

"That's great!" I said, through clenched teeth.

Yeah, it's true that I won the Ironman Triathlon in Hawaii six times and the Nice Triathlon ten times in ten starts. It's true that, when I was in full-time hard-core training, you would have to look pretty hard to find any extra fat floating around my midsection. With body fat hovering around 4 percent, I was carrying very little of what you might call excess baggage.

But when the call came, I wasn't in training anymore. My last Ironman had been two years earlier, in 1995. After retiring from competition, I wasn't as consistent with my workouts as I should have been. Let's be frank: I was getting a tad on the soft side.

I was fit enough to walk through the grocery store or take my son Mats to the beach without feeling self-conscious. But I wasn't sporting the look I'd like to have for a cover photo—especially one that would show up in mailboxes coast to coast, on every newsstand, in every convenience store, and in every airport in the country. Nope, I would have to get back into great shape—and I would have to do it *fast.*

My wife, Julie, and I huddled up as a family and set time lines, goals, and boundaries. Then

I set out to once again become the World's Fittest Man.

Nestled within this story is the essence of what can become the athletic mantra for all of us: finding a reason to arrive healthy and happy at our highest personal level of fitness. It's a call to take action on all levels to get beyond laziness, fear, rationalizations, excuses, and seemingly extraordinary circumstances that inhibit our commitment to being our best. It's a challenge to come up with goals that mean something to each of us personally—goals big enough and important enough to draw us up to the next level, then the one beyond that.

Having the shared support of others who value a life of fitness is one of the best ways to survive the obstacles that life can throw in the way of meeting those goals. It is special when people or families share a common framework of fitness. Creating things to do with that com-

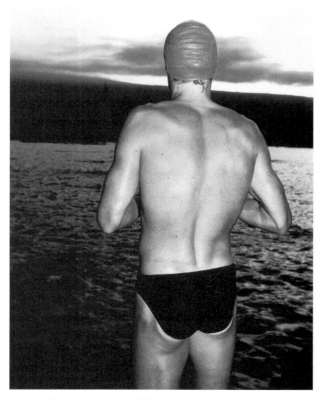

I relate the beginning of the Ironman to the beginning of your own fitness program. If you think about the magnitude of the task, it seems overwhelming. But if you take it one workout, one meal, one day at a time, you will definitely succeed.

mon ground, having goals that require the two of you to work together, makes the commitment stronger and the chance of success more likely.

I can't tell you how much training I missed when I was working out by myself. But when I made a commitment to meet people for a workout, I always made it. Old training partners reading this may call me up and say, "What do you mean? You missed that long ride in '83." So, okay, I may have been late a few times, but I did not blow them off.

Julie: The Ironwoman Mark and I got together because of the Ironman. Ironically, I did the event before he did—before we were anything more than casual acquaintances.

My introduction to the Ironman Triathlon was in 1981. It was my senior year in college as a physical education major. One rainy Saturday afternoon in February, I was curled up in front of the television, doing more watching than studying. *ABC's Wide World of Sports* came on with its classic opening footage and slogan of "the thrill of victory and the agony of defeat." The show was devoted to a crazy multisport competition set on the Big Island of Hawaii— the Ironman Triathlon. The competitors started the day with a 2.4-mile swim in the warm Hawaiian waters. Then they mounted their bikes for a 112-mile ride through the desolate lava fields on the island's dry west side. The day finished off with a 26.2-mile run, a marathon under the searing heat of a tropical sun. The sheer audacity of the distances combined with the beauty and brutality of the Big Island were compelling.

For the next hour and a half, I was completely mesmerized. Those Ironman competitors were going way beyond anything even remotely resembling my developing concept of lifestyle fitness. At the time, I was just playing around with my own personal fitness, trying to combat those freshman "dorm food" pounds that I hadn't been able to shake.

I'd been a surfer since I was fourteen, but I was hardly a jock. However, as the days passed, the Ironman lingered in my mind. It got to me in a way I couldn't put my finger on. Around

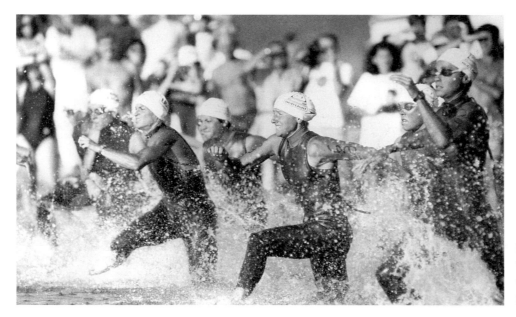

Forget about sitting on the sidelines! The best way to change your life? Plunge into fitness!

the same time, I needed to commit to a topic for my senior thesis. Those powerful images of the Hawaii Ironman and my need for a senior project coalesced and I had it. I'd research and train for the Ironman, and it would all culminate with my crossing the finish line of the next year's event.

Researching the Ironman back in 1981 was short and sweet. There was exactly one published article in *Sports Illustrated* magazine detailing the event in 1979. The rest of my project was filled in with some training concepts and physiological studies on marathon runners. The bulk of my project was theory and conjecture, with very little practical application. In other words, I used my standard approach to school, which was to wing it.

When I stepped off the plane in Hawaii the following February, I had yet to swim or ride the full distances required. To my credit, I had completed two marathons—both in the previous six weeks. Including the Ironman, I would be running three marathons in a two-month stretch. This was hardly ideal, but I was young. I thought, "So what?"

I had two weeks on the island to train before the event. In that time, I logged close to 400 miles on the bike, including one 140-miler. After that, I was confident I could go the distance.

On race morning, as I treaded water waiting for the starting gun, I remember feeling nervous, excited, and relieved all at the same time. All I hoped was to make it to the finish and to be able to graduate with my degree in physical education. I never dreamed this would be the beginning of a lifelong association with the sport of triathlon and personal fitness.

Yet that day changed my life. I would never feel the same way about myself or put the same physical limits on what I could accomplish again.

Defining Moments In 1982, Julie Moss's athletic performance at the Hawaiian Ironman Triathlon went beyond winning, beyond sport, and smashed head-on into the realm of human drama. She led the women's field after nearly ten hours of racing. As she came down to the final 400 meters, however, with the finish line banner in sight, her body simply gave out. She went from running to walking to staggering in the blink of an eye. The frailty of the human body was on display before millions as she stumbled and then fell. Like a fawn taking its first steps, she willed herself to her feet and continued on toward what would have been the biggest win of her young career.

Like a punch-drunk fighter, she was out on her feet, oblivious to the crowd massed on each side of her. She fell again and lay on the street.

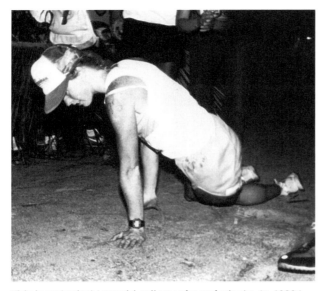

This is not what I would call my résumé photo. In 1982 I found myself leading the most important triathlon in the world with *ABC's Wide World of Sports* covering my every move. Then, about one hundred yards from the finish, my body simply ran out of gas. I walked, staggered, and then fell to the ground. Within sight of the line, I was passed and lost the lead. But in my mind I had come to Kona for only one purpose: to finish the Ironman. So I used what energy I had left to crawl the rest of the way, collapsing at the finish line while cameras zoomed in for more. It was the perfect agony-of-defeat shot for which *ABC's Wide World of Sports* has become so famous. But I am proud of what I accomplished that day. Sure, looking back, I wish I had eaten more and taken in more fluids. But I realize that my race had impact. I went as hard as I could for as long as I could and came up a tad short. After watching that show, a lot of people, including my husband-to-be Mark Allen, were motivated to get off the couch and start training for the Ironman. Just finishing, just getting to the line no matter what, became both my legacy and the Ironman mantra.

Her body had betrayed her. With less than five yards to go, the second-place woman passed her for the win. With the ABC cameras recording each moment, Julie summoned every ounce of courage and crawled toward the line. The crowd went deathly silent. Within an arm's length of the finish, she reached one hand across the line and collapsed onto her back. There was a small smile playing at the corners of her lips as she was carried to the medical tent.

Her message was clear: To win is to finish. To finish is to win. It was one of those magical moments that goes beyond competition, beyond comprehension. Julie had ignored the warning signs and had refused to give in. As millions wiped tears away from their eyes in the security of their living rooms, a young woman pushed the envelope and went way beyond the limits of what the human body is capable of.

Julie's race that day, at the age of twenty-three, inspired the growth of what had been a relatively obscure sport. Her willingness to keep going, to cross that finish line no matter what, made her special. Even though her ideal race had evaporated in the heat of the lava fields, she struck an emotional chord in every one of the millions who watched *ABC's Wide World of Sports* that day.

Mark: A Lifestyle of Fitness I was one of those many people who were deeply touched by Julie's overwhelming humanness at the end of an event that seemed to be defined by superhuman efforts.

Barely six months after watching what was a watershed moment in the sport of triathlon, I was on the start line of that incredible race. Part of me was absolutely terrified of the challenges awaiting me out there in the endless miles of the Big Island's lava fields. I don't know how I would have felt if I'd known the twists and turns my life would encounter because of this race and Julie's inspiration six months earlier.

Over the next fifteen years, I traveled the world, racing some of the fittest athletes on the planet. I married my original inspiration, Julie Moss. But more important than any of the race victories Julie and I accumulated during that time was a lifestyle of fitness and health that evolved into the fabric of our relationship with each other and with our training partners. A good day became defined by the quality of our workouts and the people we shared it with.

Surprisingly, fitness and health have become even more important in our lives since we ended serious competition. Balancing work and family only happens for us when personal health is factored in, which is why we make the time to keep our connections to our own fitness and our community of athletic friends.

Life is more complicated now, and time for working out that used to be so abundant years ago is much harder to find. But fitness is who we are and who we always hope to be. We will always have a commitment to our physical, emotional, and spiritual well-being.

Julie After his initial year in triathlons, Mark's fitness took a huge leap. At first, we were close to the same speed. Eventually, we became incompatible as side-by-side training partners, which did not mean that the motivation and support ended. It was still exciting to come home at the end of a workout day and share the stories, tell about the moments that stood out, and congratulate each other when we hit new levels of fitness.

Support and balance can come indirectly, too. The year our son Mats arrived was a tough one for me athletically. I had several failed attempts to run a fast marathon from 1991 to 1993, and by Ironman in October I was very pregnant. Forget marathoning. At that point, easy swimming had become my only exercise.

It was finally time to enjoy a supporting role for Mark, relax about my personal athletic journey, and get a new perspective. My life needed a clean slate. Mark absolved all my personal failures by capturing his fourth Hawaii Ironman title with his magnificent performance.

Julie: Joy Joy is seeing Mats standing on the end of a surfboard for the first time. Or watching him barrel down a ski hill with his buddies. It's also knowing I've put my heart and soul into preparing for a goal, then nailing it. In the past, I've picked long-term projects like doing the Ironman and running a marathon. I don't arrive at the finish overnight. The joy is proportionate to the time and energy it takes to complete it.

Emotional Benefits of Fitness Beyond the tangible, there are emotional and spiritual benefits to fitness that could be summed up by one word: *joy*. It feels good to sweat, to work out, to be physically strong. You are happier when you move your body, when you test yourself physically, when you gain resilience through the health of your body, when you push the limit on a physical level. Along the way, you discover a connection to your own power and to the life force itself. The measurement of these things is not as concrete as weight loss or a good finish time at a race. But even those definable qualities from fitness are meaningful because they increase that undeniable quality of joy.

An athletic body is a powerful thing in and of itself. It's even more amazing when it's a reflection of the joy you feel just from being alive.

Your Maximum Potential What we mean by "using fitness to its maximum potential" is using fitness to explore the intangibles. Maximum potential is going beyond just losing fat and increasing longevity. It's using exercise, racing, and higher levels of fitness to create a sense of well-being, a peace of mind.

Up the ante in your level of fitness to increase the feeling of power in your own body. Make the commitment of time and energy you need to explore greater levels of what you can do physically. It will expand the realms of possibility in all areas of your life.

What could possibly be holding you back?

One Caveat Depending on your current level of fitness, it's a good idea to get a check-up before you start an exercise program or make a significant increase in your workout load. At least 10 percent of adults in the United States have high blood pressure, and at least 50 percent have poor cholesterol levels.

Julie: Excuses Certainly there are valid excuses for not exercising. Motherhood is a valid excuse. For me, a good excuse for missing a workout is because I have something to do for my son. You need to make executive decisions on what are excuses and what are priorities, though. If your children are the priority and your baby-sitter doesn't show up, then you have to cancel your workout with your partner. That is not an excuse. That's a priority.

The excuse I try using the most often is, "At the end of a day I'm just too tired to work out." Then I think about what my priorities are. Do I want to lounge in front of the television or read a magazine for an hour, or do I want to get out the door? I try to choose the latter. I also try to schedule late workouts with a training partner for support and to have someone to vent about the day with. Once I get going, I always find the

energy. This is the happy mystery—working out can create energy to add to the end of your day.

Mark: No Excuses I probably have more excuses than the average human. To keep myself on track, I try to pick a goal that I'm scared to death to *not* be prepared for. A little, easy-to-

---

Excuse Checkers

It's time to dock your little boat of excuses. They just don't hold water anymore—and they're in danger of drowning you. Here are enough life preservers to get you safely home:

EXCUSE: *My day is so packed I don't have any big blocks of time to work out.* **REBUTTAL:** Studies have shown that three 10-minute bouts of activity produce virtually the same health benefits as a 30-minute lump.

EXCUSE: *I may not work out that much, but that's okay because I'm not fat.* **REBUTTAL:** Poor fitness is as likely to kill you as cigarette smoking.

EXCUSE: *I hate to run, and walking seems like a lame exercise.* **REBUTTAL:** Walking burns almost the same number of calories as running the same distance.

EXCUSE: *Neither my mate nor I are interested in exercise.* **REBUTTAL:** Regular exercise improves circulation, and men don't need a degree to understand the importance of blood flow to certain body parts. Regular exercise is one of several factors that can help prevent impotence.

EXCUSE: *I'm too heavy and out of shape. Exercising could be dangerous.* **REBUTTAL:** Overweight people who exercise can lower their blood pressure even if they don't lose weight.

EXCUSE: *I work out three days a week. Enough, already!* **REBUTTAL:** Expanding your investment in workout time to one and a half to two hours a day, four to six days a week, will significantly alter your body and your health, enhancing your life in many unforeseen ways.

achieve goal will not make me go into action. Try to win an Ironman? That scares me into preparing. There is no excuse large enough to keep me from being ready when I face that start line.

Mark: Professionally Fit Unlike most people, for fifteen years my job consisted of training and racing as a professional triathlete. It was my sole means of support, and many of my friends were athletes in the same position: Train all day, every day. During that period I never understood the challenge most people have to find the time for fitness in the packed life of work and family. I was in for an eye-opener in the fall of 1996, when I retired from racing.

Everything changed. Suddenly, even when the desire was there, I had a hard time just getting out the door for a run. By the fall of 1997, I had let the downhill fitness slide happen. I had become a living example of the classic excuse-making, no-workout persona—too little time, too many responsibilities.

Julie would grab the spare tire I was sporting around my midsection and give it a yank. She was training for an Ironman comeback at the age of thirty-nine and getting fitter by the day. I was going in the opposite direction. My pride was tarnished, and physically I felt rotten. Once again, Julie became my inspiration to get back at it.

My commitment was simple: Do something each day. Make the time for one workout every day and come up with whatever reason I needed to keep on track. It took several months for the rhythm to return, but it did. Now I'm no longer the master of the great excuse. And every aspect of my life works smoother because my fitness is back.

Taking Steps to Fitness A lot of people say, "Gee, I want to run a 10K. I want to run a marathon. I saw one on TV. My friends did it. How can I do that? I don't know where to start." Do not get stuck in the not-knowing. You get beyond it by taking the first step and trying. The first step will lead to the next one

and the one after that. Your body will tell you how to adjust if you listen to it. Your body is your wisest guide.

The important thing is to key in on the word *steps*, because reaching any goal is a process of steps, not leaps. Take one after another after another. It is like the transformation from rosebud to rose. It takes place over weeks. At any one time, you might not feel an increase in fitness. Tuesday will probably feel just like Monday. You might not be able to feel the difference you made in your body and energy level. It may feel the same from this Monday to the next one. But stick with it. Getting in shape takes time. For a young person, going from sedentary to in-shape takes about three to five months. For an older person, the same progress takes from six months to a year.

Are you working out? No? Take a walk. Start with ten minutes. Anybody can find a spare ten minutes. Ask yourself: How did that feel? Feel like you did a little something? It should. It's more than you did before. Want more? Do it again tomorrow. And the next day. At the very minimum, you should be walking briskly ten minutes a day, six days a week.

After two weeks, increase the time to fifteen minutes. Just walking, but keeping a steady pace, holding your back straight and moving your arms. Every two weeks, up the time by five minutes. The next thing you know, you are walking for thirty minutes six days a week, and you're spending an extra five minutes stretching afterward. You might be the one others look up to as motivation or intimidation!

At this point, you're ready to up the ante. The easiest way to do this is to jog. Depending on your level of fitness, this might even be your starting point. If you haven't run for a few years, try alternating five minutes of running with five minutes of walking for your full thirty minutes. Gradually increase the run time while decreasing the walk time. Eventually, you'll be running for thirty minutes. Now you're ready to add strength training twice a week and a longer, slow run once a week. If you're pressed for time, skip your run on gym days. By this time, you'll be used to spending thirty to forty-five minutes a day working out, and your weekly day off will start to feel odd. Meanwhile, you'll find that you feel better, sleep better, and look better than ever.

The first step starts with a goal, a dream of transformation, and the idea that you want to experience something different. The next step and the ones after that continue with the support of your mate, your workout community, the help of your training partners, and the personally good feelings you have when you reach new milestones.

Mark: In the Beginning Before I started doing triathlons in 1982, I ran hardly more than a handful of times in a year. It was a completely foreign experience for me. I felt awkward, like Bambi on ice. Every step took a huge mental effort. My body hurt every single time. This was not the nirvana of exercise I had been told about. It was the discomfort of doing something foreign that I was not good at. I did not like it—at first!

There were many points during that first year when I just wanted to hang it up. But the intrigue of my goal, to race the Ironman, kept luring me. And if I was ever going to complete the Ironman, I was going to have to learn how to run.

So I stuck with it. Progress wasn't easy physically or mentally. I always felt as if I were one step away from being injured. The concept of pleasure did not even enter my mind when I was out there doing it. Painfully, I worked my mileage up over time from 2 miles—where I started out—to about 6 to 8 miles on my consistent runs and over 13 on my longer ones.

Slowly my body began to adapt. The change was so slow, in fact, that I didn't notice the runs were starting to get easier. Eventually, the 8-milers became more enjoyable than those first 2-milers.

All of a sudden I went through a barrier, a doorway, that I hadn't known existed. Running had required a lot of conscious effort, but one day I passed through to a place where my mind was free. It felt easy and totally enjoyable. It was a real, concrete sense of proficiency.

I had moments when running was enjoyable before I reached proficiency. And afterward there were times where it required conscious

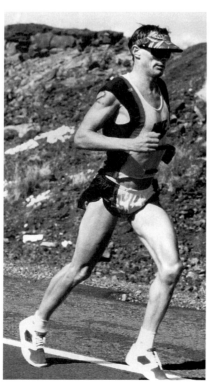
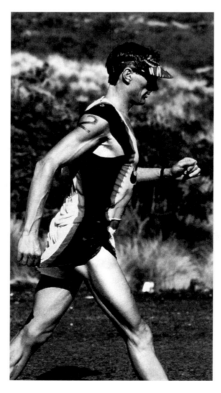
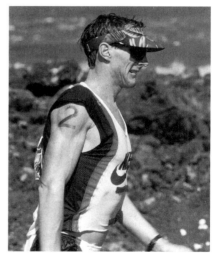

During the 1987 Ironman I was leading late in the run (far left) before my body gave out and I was forced to walk (near left and above). I ended up in second place, but I also ended up in the hospital with internal bleeding. Not one of my best days.

thought to keep going. But the bulk of the time, from that day on I loved running!

But it took time.

I've said "I'll start Monday," countless times. The beginning is the most difficult step, next to the final step before it's over. The preparation for the first step is important, but it does not actually count as the first step. Buying the new running shoes and outfits does not actually count as a workout. The first step is actually going out and doing some sort of physical activity, and then carry on from there.

Julie: Beginnings

Beginnings can be tough, but they are hopeful times when you set goals and shoot for the moon. Beginnings also give you a chance to prioritize, to figure out what might be helpful in attaining the goal, like improving your diet, getting a coach, seeking a training group, working on flexibility. It's a time to try new approaches.

Once your plans are mapped out, it's time to dig in and start taking your exercise program one day at a time. What you accomplish tomorrow is just as important as what you accomplish five months from now. It's patience and consistency in small, steady steps.

Overcoming Negative Images, Thoughts, and Patterns

Living your greatest level of health and fitness requires looking beyond the physical realm. The mechanics of training are just some of the ingredients in the recipe for ultimate health. Complete success depends on a few other elements. Whether the goal is losing fifty pounds or racing the Eco-Challenge, there are thoughts, patterns of behavior, and self-images that can hold you back.

How do you see yourself, your body, and your potential? "I'm not an athlete!" "I'm too old!" "I'm too fat!" Or "I just don't have what it takes to race well." These negative self-images are like invisible corrosives to your willpower and determination to transform yourself.

The talk that goes on inside you ends up defining the world you exist in. Positive thoughts will set you free. Negative ones put invisible fences around your potential. Holding on to your current body image can prevent the desired body image from appearing. To really enjoy success at fitness, you have to overcome negative thoughts and images. And, as hard as it can be to hear the truth from them, your partner can be the best resource for helping you see where your patterns of behavior and internal images are limiting you instead of helping you accomplish your goals.

Julie: Body Image

Changing my body image is one of the biggest benefits I received from being a competitive athlete. Now I place importance on what my body can do rather than how it looks. The images in fashion magazines are no longer my goal. Ironically, the more I can do physically, the better I like the way my body looks.

That's not to say that physical beauty and fitness aren't a dynamic combination. For example, we have the good fortune to be friendly with the übercouple Gabby Reese and Laird Hamilton. Gabby is a six-foot-three-inch supermodel and pro volleyball player who is even more gorgeous in person than in print or on television. Her husband is an extreme surfer and all-around water man who has one of the best male bodies around. With their looks and fitness, they could be very intimidating. But what I see and relate to in them is that they are another couple who shares a passion for fitness, and I enjoy hanging out with them.

For most of my adult life, my self-image has been totally defined through my association with triathlons and an athletic lifestyle. This has allowed me to avoid many of the pitfalls facing women in our society concerning physical perfectionism. Through athletics, I've adopted a positive image that feels healthy and well balanced.

> *There is no disadvantage to being healthy, and there are a lot of advantages. It is a matter of committing yourself to being healthy.*

Don't Hold Yourself Back In many ways, giving up habits that hold you back from reaching your physical goals is much easier than actually getting out there and tackling a fitness program. Say one of your bad habits is eating too much sugar. To give it up, simply don't eat it—don't buy it, don't have it around the house, don't look at it in the office or on a menu. A fitness program, on the other hand, requires *action,* which means finding the motivation and time, and then actually getting out there and doing it.

Try to find ways to incorporate movement into your lifestyle. Think about it. It can be as easy as parking at the far end of the parking lot. Or:

- Walk to work. Walk home from work.

- When you get home from work, go for a jog with your significant other and discuss the events of the day. Bicycle to your friend's house for a visit.

- Organize a workout group with the parents in your neighborhood. Take turns watching all the kids while the rest of the group goes for a run, ride, or whatever.

- Instead of sitting and gossiping while your kids are at play group, bring some hand weights and do a strength workout while you're watching your heir run about the park.

- When your family gets together, do it outdoors. Bring baseball, football, or Frisbee equipment—and use it!

- Encourage your roommate to exercise. Be helpful and supportive. Then go with her.

Search your mind and your life for motivation to work out. Associate with people who are physically active. Think positive, in terms of "I will" and "I can." There are also motivational tricks you can play, like:

- Pay yourself to work out longer. Think of something you really want, and paste a picture of it on a jar. Put five bucks in the jar for every twenty minutes you work out until you've reached your goal. Then think of something else you want.

- Invite your biggest rival to work out with you.

- Tell everybody you know that you're going to work out this afternoon or tomorrow morning. Or enter a marathon and tell everybody you know. Stick your neck out.

It's not hard. You just have to think about what you normally do, and add motion to it.

Fitness and Family For many people, starting a family means the end of their fitness regime. Increased responsibilities—along with some outmoded assumptions about what family life is all about—take their toll. Yet, when babies are very young, it's quite easy to incorporate them into your workout. Use a Baby Jogger or a backpack carrier to take them with you on your run or bicycle ride. Set up a weight bench in the house and keep the kids nearby, sleeping or playing in a basket or stroller. As they get older, you can leave them with a baby-sitter while you work out (baby-sitters aren't only for evenings on the town!). Or they can play with their friends down the street while you get a run in.

If you start with the assumption that you can work the kids into your fitness plan, you'll do it. Before long, they'll become a part of that fitness lifestyle, running and playing with you, cheering for you at races. It's time spent together that you'll always treasure.

Julie: Becoming a Family By early 1993, we were wholeheartedly in the baby-making business. The ticking of my biological clock drowned the voices inside me that wanted to set another big athletic goal. Mats was conceived in the spring of that year and I found a whole new approach to fitness. My past personal fitness rules no longer applied. While Mark's road was well paved from years of experience, mine was now completely new.

At every turn, I faced new physical adventures and new emotional challenges. I was able to redefine pregnancy fitness on a daily basis. It was a blissful time in our lives. I stood at the finish line at the Ironman that year, waiting to greet Mark en route to a record fifth consecutive Ironman title. I let my greatly expanded waistline define my athletic goals for the moment and learned to enjoy my partner's success. Our son Mats was born one month later.

As a new mother, getting back into shape was my second priority. It seemed logical somehow that it should take an equal nine months to get back into shape. This proved to be pretty accurate, especially for a nursing mother. The key to my post-pregnancy fitness was my Baby Jogger. Mats and I entered our first 5K in March, with Mats edging me out for the win by the length of our Jogger. In less than two years, we wore the treads off the Jogger's tires.

Mark skipped the Ironman in 1994, but we returned as a family for his final race in Hawaii in 1995. Waiting for Mark to finish while holding Mats, I felt so complete. We were about to share Mark's Ironman victory as a family for the first time. Seeing Mark cross the line and reaching to give Mats and me the kiss we'd waited over eight hours for is a memory that will last me a lifetime. Mark recorded his sixth Ironman victory and ended his Ironman career all in that moment. Our life as a family was about to become a clean slate.

Now we have a child we can inspire. Mats likes to run. He picks it up from watching us. He started running and I think we explained a few things about pacing, to slow down if you want to last a while. The first few times we went running, he went out too fast and walked home, but the last time he ran over thirty minutes and only took a few breaks to look for feathers and flowers. Actually, Mats asks to go running more and more, and what was going to be a warm-up for Mark ends up being Mats's run.

Mats: Family When you are out racing a race, you should never forget about your family. That's the most important thing.

2 Defining Your Fitness

itness doesn't have just one definition. It has a million. What fitness looks like in the mind of a javelin thrower trying to make an Olympic team will be very different from the picture a ballerina has when she is planning to perform onstage. And those two images and definitions of fitness will be different from the one a sedentary forty-year-old will come up with. Our bodies and our goals will define what fitness means to us.

Fitness also has an ever-changing definition as your body and ability change. A mile walk twice a week may seem like an eternity and a supreme effort today. Five years from now, after logging in at the lifelong fitness club, that same person may be feeling cheated if he or she doesn't get in 5 to 10 miles a day every day of the week.

Mark I used to work out every day, all day. If I couldn't get in at least three hours a day, it just didn't seem worth the bother. Then Mats was born. Sleepless nights took the edge off my competitive desire, and I was exhausted most of the time. A lot of days, it would be near sunset before I was able to consider rallying for a workout. By that time, there wasn't enough time left in the day to make my three-hour minimum.

Days would go by without workouts. My fitness skidded into the garbage can of my self-imposed limits. Finally, the lightbulb went on and I realized fifteen to twenty minutes of *something* was better than no minutes of anything. Eventually, I got in shape, and Mats started sleeping through the night. It all started when I worked out with the time I had at the fitness level I had, instead of where I wanted to be or thought I should be.

Mats: Kids' Fitness Pick up some heavy coconuts or rocks. When swimming, do laps with your arms only—no kicking—if you want to get your arms exercised. When running, go the same pace until you get close to the finish, then start running fast. The longer you run, the slower you should go, and the shorter, the faster. I ran a 5K. I like running with Mommy.

Julie: Success As a wife and mother, I can state unequivocally: Success is getting out the door.

A New Reality As little as two centuries ago (and even today in many cultures), fitness was a byproduct of living. Cavemen and -women had to use their bodies to stay alive. A sedentary Neanderthal was probably a dead Neanderthal. Shopping in nature's grocery store required a much greater expenditure of calories than hopping in the car, going to the market, and rolling the cart down the aisles. If you look at life from this perspective, things are much easier for us than they were for our ancestors.

By other standards, our lives are extremely difficult. It is not easy to live in a way that balances our need for exercise, rest, and regeneration time spent just hanging out and joking with family and friends. In the modern world, achieving even modest levels of physical fitness requires *creating* physical activity and carving time out of jammed lifestyles to do it. Fitness is no longer a byproduct of our existence.

There are many realities. One is the reality of your life as seen through the eyes of a fairly biased expert, which is *you*. Based on your assessment, life may seem good or not. You may feel in shape, or not. You may or may not think there is enough time and energy available for you to contemplate starting a workout program. You could be paralyzed by the prospect of having to stick to one for any length of time. No matter what your assessment of your lifestyle, with all its positives and its faults, no matter how accurate or inaccurate your assessment, it is very real—because you believe it is.

There is another reality. It affects your life regardless of how much or how little importance you place on it. This is the natural world, the reality that you are a biological machine with a spirit that, like any other machine, requires proper maintenance, upgrading, and testing to keep it doing the job it was built to do.

An optimal experience of life happens when these two realities become the same. Taking care of your body helps improve the health and function of your mind. Positive thoughts in turn help keep your body healthy. Choosing good food over junk, replacing stress with rest, and working your body as well as your mind all add up to developing a positive relationship with the reality that exists beyond your own personal one.

A natural existence requires using not only your *mental* powers but also your *physical* ones—your body. Look at your life. Is the energy usage all mental? Energetically, this would be like eating only one food. Adding physical activity to the mix puts variety into the energy of your life. It brings your whole being into harmony. It can actually add energy to you.

> *One research study shows that with thirty minutes a day of exercise, people increase their work output by 15 percent.*

Lifetime Health, Just 2,000 Calories a Week The bottom line here is activity level and your body's composition. For activity, burning 2,000 calories a week through exercise is the magic number that research says will extend your life the most. A Stanford University study of over 16,000 Harvard alumni found that men who burned 2,000 calories a week—the equivalent of about 3 miles of brisk walking a day—had 39 percent less risk of developing coronary artery disease. In terms of weekly exercise time, this comes out to about three and a half hours.

We're talking about burning calories, which means elevating your heart rate. Many sports don't qualify. Tennis and golf are enjoyable, but three and a half hours on the court does not equate to three and a half hours of cardiovascular exercise. You can only count the amount of time your heart rate is elevated and your body is in motion.

Composition Next up is body composition. If you are carrying too much fat inside, regardless of what your shape is on the outside, you could be shortening your life. And *composition* is the key word here. Not all thin-looking people are lean or healthy. Nor are all large people anywhere close to having a body composition that is unhealthy in terms of excess fat.

Here is a simple formula you can use to determine where you are on this scale. It is called the Body Mass Index (BMI), which is a way of measuring your body weight in relation to your height. Take your body weight in kilograms (1 kilo equals 2.2 pounds) and divide it by your height in meters (1 meter equals 3.28 feet). This gives your BMI. A body mass of 26 or higher is considered overweight, and means that—even though the contours may be good-looking— some attention needs to be given to changing the body composition through exercise to decrease fat and increase muscle mass. (Note: body builders and other athletes with a very large amount of muscle mass can actually have a BMI above 26.) The chart below has the BMI calculated for a variety of heights and weights. Just find your height (in inches) on the left, and go to your weight (in pounds) to the right of that. Then at the bottom of that column is your BMI.

Body Mass Index

HEIGHT (INCHES)	BODY WEIGHT (POUNDS)							OVERWEIGHT					OBESE				
58	91	96	100	105	110	115	119	124	129	134	138	143	148	153	158	162	167
59	94	99	104	109	114	119	124	128	133	138	143	148	153	158	163	168	173
60	97	102	107	112	118	123	128	133	138	143	148	153	158	163	168	174	179
61	100	106	111	116	122	127	132	137	143	148	153	158	164	169	174	180	185
62	104	109	115	120	126	131	126	142	147	153	158	164	169	175	180	186	191
63	107	113	118	124	130	135	141	146	152	158	163	169	175	180	186	191	197
64	110	116	122	128	134	140	145	151	157	163	169	174	180	186	192	197	204
65	114	120	126	132	138	144	150	156	162	168	174	180	186	192	198	204	210
66	118	124	130	136	142	148	155	161	167	173	179	186	192	198	204	210	216
67	121	127	134	140	146	153	159	166	72	178	185	191	198	204	211	217	223
68	125	131	138	144	151	158	164	171	177	184	190	197	203	210	216	223	230
69	128	135	142	149	155	162	169	176	182	189	196	203	209	216	223	230	236
70	132	139	146	153	160	167	174	181	188	195	202	209	216	222	229	236	243
71	136	143	150	157	165	172	179	186	193	200	208	215	222	229	236	242	250
72	140	147	154	162	169	177	184	191	199	206	213	221	228	235	242	250	258
73	144	151	159	166	174	182	189	197	204	212	219	227	235	242	250	257	265
74	148	155	163	171	179	186	194	202	210	218	225	233	241	249	256	264	272
75	152	160	168	176	184	192	200	208	216	224	232	240	248	256	264	272	279
76	156	164	172	180	189	197	205	213	221	230	238	246	254	263	271	279	287
BMI	19	20	21	22	23	24	25	26	27	28	29	30	31	32	33	34	35

To determine your body mass index (BMI) find your height (in inches) along the left column. Then follow it over to your weight (in pounds) to the right. At the bottom of that column is a number that indicates your BMI. A BMI of 24 or less is considered ideal, a BMI of 25 to 29 is considered to be overweight, and a BMI of 30 to 35 is considered to be obese. It should be noted that someone can actually have a BMI over 24 and still be very healthy if that number is skewed up because of a large amount of lean muscle mass, as is the case for a lot of body builders and elite athletes.

Start From Where You Are . . . Right Now Regardless of your personal definition of fitness and what you are after from training, there are four basic elements that everyone in every sport at every level of fitness uses to improve from where they are *right now*. Those elements are *strength*, *endurance*, *flexibility*, and *diet*. They are the golden tools that can take off fifty pounds, lower cholesterol, increase longevity, and decrease stress. They are also the keys that can get you in the shape it takes to win an Ironman. The only difference will be the amount of time you actually spend working out and the workout activities you will choose to accomplish your goals.

Strength

- Are you under thirty years old?

- Are you getting the race results you are after on a strict diet of cardiovascular (aerobic) exercise?

- Do you actually use that health club card to lift weights twice a week?

- Do you have the same strength you had five years ago?

- Does that active vacation leave you sore and needing another vacation to recover from it?

- If you couldn't afford the Skycap, could you actually carry your own luggage?

If your answer is no to any of these questions, it is probably time to get it together and get on the strength program outlined in Chapter 6.

Endurance (Aerobic) Exercise The key here is finding exercise that elevates your heart rate for a sustained period of time. If your goal is weight loss and/or longevity, there is no way around it: You have to move your body. If you are a competitor at heart, again, there is no way around it. Aerobic fitness helps all sports.

Here are a few tests and tips to help take you to the next level.

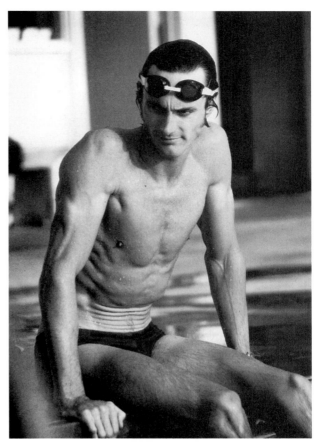

Okay, so I bore a passing resemblance to a skeletal anatomy chart in the early 1980s. Over time, though, I learned the value of weight training and the need to build strength, especially as you age.

- Does climbing stairs leave you breathless? If so, walk.

- Are your kids running circles around you? If so, run.

- Does it take more than two minutes to get your heart rate below 100 when you stop exercising? If so, kick the aerobic program up a few notches, but do it in the way we recommend in Chapter 5. Not all aerobic exercise is created equal.

- If two days of exercise help you feel better, try three, then four, then more.

- Pick a measurable quantity in the aerobic sport of your choice—laps, distance, time. Time it, measure it, do it at your best level. Then dedicate yourself to improving through increased fitness over the next three months. Then go back and repeat the process. Measurable improvement is always motivating.

If you want to improve your endurance, read Chapters 6 and 8.

Flexibility With age comes inflexibility in your muscles and tendons. This makes you more likely to have joint pain, back pain, and frequent injuries to muscles when you do work out. Along with lack of strength, lack of flexibility is one of the main reasons for sudden spasms and injury in older people from sideways twisting motions. But, like just about every other physical sign of aging, there is something we can do about it.

Here's the test: When was the last time you stretched for more than about three minutes? If it wasn't within the last week, it's time to stretch. If you can't remember, it's *really* time to stretch. If you never have, you don't know what you are missing. See our program in Chapter 7.

Diet All the workouts in the world won't get you to your ultimate level of health if you don't support them with a balanced diet. We all know that, but what does it mean?

Here's the diet test, and it holds for all meals. Look at your plate and see what's on it.

- Is there a source of a complete protein?
- Can you see monounsaturated fat or other vegetable fat?
- Are the carbohydrates from whole grains, legumes, fruits, vegetables?

If the answer is no to any of these questions, check out the information on diet and nutrition later in this book. If you don't know whether the answer is yes or no, read Chapter 9, make a conscious effort to improve your diet, then ask the questions again.

Mark: Value Anything that brings more energy and a better balance to your life has value. And not just the quick fixes that some people are looking for. I'm talking about the more lasting ones, like real health, real balance between our bodies, hearts, and spirits.

Total Fitness: Body, Attitude, Spirit

The physical benefits of moving your body include weight loss, strength gain, and a general transformation in physical appearance. Other benefits are less tangible, but no less real. After working out for ten to twenty minutes, you enter a regenerative state not only for your body, but also for your mind and spirit. You simply feel better. It is one of the addictive, healing qualities of exercise.

Just as important as working your body is making sure you have a healthy attitude, strong spirit, and joyful heart. They are all intertwined. Look at the number of cigarette smokers who defy research and live to a ripe old age. Zest for life and an overwhelming feeling of joy just being here on earth can overcome even significant health hazards.

Then there are the health nuts who die in their fifties. Stresses, anger, sadness, lack of appreciation for life . . . they'll do you in quicker than cigarettes.

You want to be happy? Here are some basics:

- **Work out regularly,** which by our definition means doing some form of exercise every day. Exercise your heart, your muscles, and your flexibility. Life is less of a challenge if physical strength and endurance are not limiting factors.

- **Make smart food choices.** Choose foods that look something like they did in nature. The less they look like they did when they came off the vine, the more processed they are and the worse they will be for you. Diet is as important as exercise in maintaining good health.

- **Rest. Yes, rest.** We all need it, but very few people get enough of it. Eight hours a night is recommended, but the actual number that will keep you sharp all day and not feeling exhausted at bedtime can range from six to ten.

- **Regenerate vigorously.** Take an active vacation, spending your time outside the hotel room—it's easy if you are in shape.

• **Regenerate quietly.** This can take many forms, including a spiritual practice, meditation, even reading. Just do something that allows your mind to let go. Simply *be.* Take a moment, a day, a week away from the responsibilities, thoughts, and patterns of living that drag your energy and enthusiasm down. A moment of internal quiet can balance days of racing through life.

Mark I learned in my triathlon career that happiness and race results, although often linked, were not the key to being completely fulfilled in my life. There were many races that I won that didn't have a very lasting effect on my sense of well-being. Feeling physically fit, staying healthy, and racing fast was just part of the equation. Beyond that was having balance between the time I spent training (work time for me), time with Julie, and eventually, time with Mats.

There was also that component of being an integral part of nature. Gazing into my computer screen is just not the same as gazing at a sunset. Listening to my answering machine does not have quite the same balancing effect on my system as listening to the ocean or a stream. And the sixty-watt energy-saver bulb just doesn't replace the sunshine. A big reason why Julie and I work out now is to enjoy the outdoors in a participatory way. We trail-run, ski, hike, and surf

---

Scare Tactics

A beer today or a bonbon tomorrow will not kill you. Overdo it all the time, and you are dead meat at an early age. Miss your walk on Tuesday, then blow off weights on Wednesday, and no one will know but your empty logbook. Keep it up for a year and you will transform yourself, but in the wrong direction. There is always an excuse, but how many are as important as making sure you are around to make another one tomorrow?

You've probably heard all the reasons why you should work out, both the positive benefits and negatives you have to look forward to if you don't. But just in case they aren't on the tip of your tongue, here's a refresher course:

• Experts have estimated that as many as 250,000 deaths a year in the United States, about 12 percent of the total, are attributable to a lack of physical activity.

• Roughly one quarter of American adults remain sedentary.

• If you don't act to prevent it, as you age you lose about half a pound of muscle each year, and gain about one and a half pounds of fat. That's two pounds a year in the wrong direction.

• Twenty-two percent of Americans are adequately active, 54 percent inadequately active, and 24 percent completely sedentary. (*Adequate* is defined as 30 minutes throughout the day of moderately intense activity most days of the week.)

• Body fat plays a role in health, but when it comes to the risk of disease, the most important fat is intra-abdominal fat—the fat that hunkers beneath your abdominals and surrounds your internal organs. Fat on the gut is a direct sign that there is also a good layer of insulation building up around your heart and in your veins.

• According to the National Institute on Aging, nearly a third of Americans over the age of seventy-five can't climb stairs.

• In the absence of exercise, your heart's ability to pump blood drops an average of 58 percent between the ages of twenty-five and eighty-five.

• Studies have shown that being 10 percent overweight decreases a man's life expectancy by 11 percent.

• The more muscles you involve in an exercise that can sustain a raised heart rate, the more you stress your cardiovascular system, which is precisely why you won't find duckpin bowling and checkers at the top of the aerobic curve.

• Obesity increases the risk of getting asthma by three times. Obesity is defined as 35 percent overweight.

ere are a few positives for exercise:

- Shed half a pound a week, and in a year you've lost twenty-six pounds.

- People who exercise have lower intra-abdominal fat. Exercise not only makes you leaner on the outside; it makes you leaner on the inside—where, in terms of health, it matters the most.

- You'll lose an average of one point off both your systolic and diastolic blood pressure for every two pounds you lose.

- Ride a bike for thirty minutes at a moderate pace and you'll burn roughly 300 calories. Eat a six-ounce serving of French fries and you ingest 540 calories.

- Studies have shown that regular exercise can clear memory blocks, improve short-term memory, and enhance creativity—handy skills in a world where most of us survive by our wits.

- Exercise can reverse all of the biomarkers of aging. This includes improving eyesight, lower-ing cholesterol, increasing hormone levels, and reversing bone density loss.

- The negative effects of some forms of arthritis can be virtually eliminated through exercise and flexibility work.

- Studies have shown that forty minutes of exercise can lower stress levels for up to three hours. A brisk ten-minute walk can relieve tension and make you feel more energetic for up to two hours.

- Exercise increases arterial flexibility, so your heart doesn't have to work as hard to pump blood through your body. In a single day, a conditioned heart might beat 50,000 fewer times than an ill-conditioned heart.

Last but not least, consider the people in your life whom you love and the things you love to do: your wife or husband, children, close friends, walking on a warm spring day, skiing fresh powder, a quick game of hoops, the freedom of dance. They are all worth staying fit for.

very vigorously. But then we stop and just soak in the beauty of places no tour bus can get to.

Common Knowledge Everyone knows they should eat a balanced diet that comes from fresh food. We all feel how exercise can reduce the amount of stress we deal with. Most people have tried at least a few times to incorporate these two things into their lives. But to a lot of people this formula sounds like a recipe for sainthood. Most who try don't stick with it.

Those are the facts. The question is, *why?*

There are as many rationalizations for avoiding fitness as there are people who adopt unhealthy options for their lives. See if any of the following fit you during periods when you wander away from fitness, food choice, and lifestyle habits that help you stay there:

- Working out just never feels good. I'm always sore, tired, and grumpy from my workouts.

- We have kids, I have a job, and it's either time with my family or time working out. I choose my family.

- My husband (or wife or significant other) just isn't into exercise, and I don't want to go alone.

- I've been working out for a year and I don't see any change. Exercise just doesn't do anything for me.

- I ran a marathon three years ago. I have done my athletic thing. I don't need it anymore.

- I gave up sugar for a month and only lost two pounds. It's not worth the sacrifice.

- I got great results for a while, but then I got bored and, well, two days off turned into two years.

- I feel fine just the way I am. I don't think I really need to do anything about my current level of fitness (or lack thereof). Yeah, I'd like to get rid of fifteen pounds, but I'm too old to ever get down to that level again.

• I'm not a machine. You can't expect me to stick with exactly what I *should* do all the time.

Each of these rationales is more than enough to put the brakes on your fitness program. But none of them takes into account the larger picture. Maybe you just need a new perspective. It may be enough to take the negative sting out of these and other reasons for not working out and place fitness back within the realm of the attainable for real humans with real lives.

Fitness on the Job Sitting behind a desk can stagnate your body's energy. Everyone has felt this. Working out converts any sedentary energy, or even better, any toxic stress energy, into positive mental and metabolic energy. It is life-giving to breathe air into your body and sweat out the parts of the day you don't want to hold on to.

The statistics show it. People who are healthier-looking get hired first. But, looks aside, a lot of jobs require a certain level of health. If you are less healthy or overweight, statistics show you are likely to have more sick days and lower productivity than someone who is healthier. Some bean counter is going to note that.

A company in Detroit put a health facility in its plant and gave its workers the option of getting off work at four thirty P.M. to work out for half an hour or sticking it out at their job until five P.M. Those who opted to get off work at four-thirty and work out were sick less often and had higher productivity than their non-workout counterparts.

Developing Your Muscle Memory Imagine you are an archer. Initially, every time you pull the bow back and aim, there is a conscious process that goes on; raise the tip, lower the tip, sight, aim, pull, release. As your proficiency increases, the movement—even very precise movements—becomes second nature and you don't have to think about it. It's sometimes called *muscle memory.*

It's the same in golf. At first you go through a major conscious checklist before you tee off. How far back do I take the club? Is my left arm straight? Keep my eye on the ball. Eventually, each of the elements becomes second nature. Only then does it become an integrated process.

Taken individually, there are so many things to think about you cannot process them all at the same time. But as your proficiency increases, all those things link together into one fluid action. Then it can become an enjoyable activity. It's the same for running, cycling, or any form of exercise. Once you reach that point, the time you spend working out is not only helping your body, it can become quiet time for your mind as well.

Mark: Inspiration Earlier this year, I was working on a speech relating what I had learned in triathlons to the world of business. I knew the first few minutes of the speech might be the only time the audience was listening, so it had to be good. But I had a problem: I could not figure out how to open the thing. I had ideas about the middle and the end, but I had to start at the beginning.

The video! I'll show the video. Then what? How the heck could I get from the video to the introduction? I was stuck.

So I went for a run, even though I was tired and not very into it. The first five or ten minutes were terrible. I felt as if I weighed twice my normal weight and was double my real age. Finally, I warmed up, and I was no longer conscious of the fact that I was running. My mind began to wander its way through some of my experiences at the Ironman in Hawaii. All of a sudden, it was clear. *Boom!* I saw the bridge that connected the video to the beginning and the next race highlight clip that would get me into the meat of the presentation. It was suddenly clear that there was no guarantee that I could win every single time I raced. But I could give my best possible performance. I had tools that enabled me to do that, and sharing those tools was what the talk was about, helping other people reach their best performance as often as possible.

Part of the joy of working out for me is reaching this state of flow. I try to pick places that are visually nice to exercise in. Some are just familiar places. Some are safe. Some are beautiful.

Most are chosen because it's the only place I can think of to go.

The Fitness Bank Every time you go out and move your body, there is a benefit. An hour of aerobic work burns about 700 calories or the equivalent of one fifth of a pound of fat, and will take you $\frac{1}{365}$ closer to your goal for the year. Just like saving money, a percentage of all workouts will go into your fitness bank account. The rest goes to the fitness IRS. It sort of disappears into thin air.

If you work out for a week, you won't be able to take the next one off and maintain the entire benefit of those workouts. But some will linger inside your body, which is where the fitness bank is located. A percentage of those workouts will be stored in your fitness account. And when you start up again, the curve back up to where you left off will be quicker because of it. It takes roughly a day to get back to where you were for every day you took off.

Over time, you reach a critical mass at the fitness bank. You've finally made enough deposits to get your body and fitness to your goal level. Once you are there, it's time to celebrate. Keeping your body at that level is so much easier than the work it took to get there. This level of personal fitness is like finally earning and saving enough money in your investment portfolio that now all you need to do is add small maintenance amounts to live quite comfortably.

Reaching Critical Mass There are breakthrough points in workouts where time and distance pass off to pleasure and freedom. This is when there are no more bad workouts. Some may be better than others, but within each one there always seems to be something positive and enjoyable. Critical mass is when smart choices in diet and consistency in training outweigh bad habits and lack of attention to your body. It's when fitness is no longer something those other people do. You have become one of them.

You know you've reached critical mass when you look in the mirror and see your body below the neck. It's when you get grumpy because you missed a workout instead of getting in a bad mood because your workout is coming up. It's when you realize you haven't looked at the scale once in the past two weeks, but you've been working out anyway.

Critical mass is when working out becomes your play. Anyone can achieve this—you don't have to be in pro-athlete shape with a model's body.

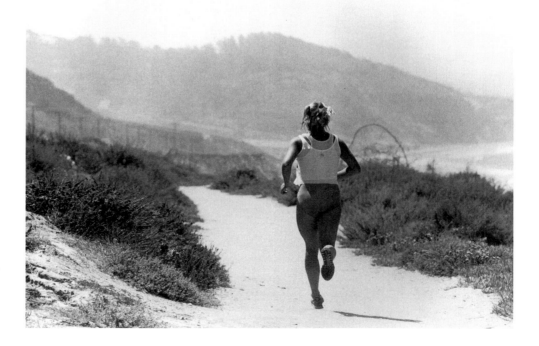

There is nothing better than your favorite running shoes and your favorite trail.

Boredom and Reality: Why We Quit When We Are Fit You may have been there once, but it slipped away. Something happened and your relationship to fitness shifted. Maybe you got bored after the initial excitement of quick results and a new training program. Hope turned into reality, and the newness became sameness. An impressive string of workouts broke. Now the only streak you are trying to keep intact is the current one of being able to keep all your clients happy, even though it's costing you your personal health.

Let's back up to the boredom. Motivation comes easily when there is progress, change, and shifts in body composition. It can slack off when you approach the limit of what will be accomplished at your current level of working out. There's nothing like losing twenty pounds in twenty weeks to keep you waking up early to meet your training buddies. It can get tough when the last five pounds take just as many months to melt away.

This is reality. There is a limit to the quick progress. There is a limit to the ultimate form your body and its health will take. And when you get there, that's the time to celebrate and congratulate yourself by making choices that maintain what you were after when you started out. That's also the point when it's easy to give up. Put that weight back on—that will motivate you again. *Or* keep it off and surrender gleefully to a lifestyle of fitness that stabilizes you there.

Staying Young People who have never experienced physical health and physical activity don't know what they are missing. They think those aches, pains, and lack of energy are just a normal part of aging. They are not!

Combining aerobic activity and weight training reverses the loss of mass in both bones and lean muscle, which happens if you don't use those muscles. Exercise also keeps hormone levels up at youthful levels and helps improve eyesight. Exercise won't keep you living forever, but it will increase your longevity and the quality of your life during the years you are here.

Aging is about discovering subtle layers of better management of your resources, of learning from your mistakes. Then you become like the old guy on the other side of the tennis net who economizes his motion. Now maybe you can't run a thirty-six-minute 10K, but you can still get out there and jog around your neigh-

> *Exercise elevates the body's levels of epinephrine and endorphins, chemicals associated with sensations of contentment and well-being.*

borhood. You can go beyond what you think you can personally do no matter what your age. When you are so dead tired and you go out anyway and find that you feel great as you run—it makes you realize how you are revitalized simply by moving your body.

Julie: Turning Forty Turning forty really got me to focus on my vision of the future. Rather than adopting a totally new lifestyle, I thought about how I could maintain my strength for the next forty years. It's less about competition and more about health. It's a shift from attaining to maintaining a strong, agile body. I will always be competitive, but my focus has shifted to the love of participating.

Diet and Fitness There are no bad foods. Your body can use just about any food when it's eaten in its natural state and in properly sized portions. Food only becomes your enemy when you refine and alter natural foods or dine on them in grossly inappropriate amounts.

We live in an eating culture. It's probably the primary activity you share with your families and friends. Christmas, Hanukkah, Thanksgiving, birthdays, office parties, dinners out, a date with your mate . . . the list never ends. Even noneating occasions are really food feasts. What would Superbowl Sunday be without four hours of gorging on a spread of snacks and alcohol?

You usually have at most one opportunity a day to work out. You have at least three, if not six to ten, opportunities to *eat* during the same period. It's easy to see why diets are so popular. With every bite you take, it can feel like you're doing something positive for your health.

Because there are so many opportunities to eat during a day, the food you consume plays a significant factor in your overall health. How you choose to eat will have a profound influence on either supporting or destroying all the work you are doing by exercising. Eating smarter is the key to using food to your advantage!

The first step in making better choices in your eating habits is to have an understanding of what fuels and repairs your body. This knowledge will keep you on track, consistently

One pound of stored fat is equal to 3,500 calories. Eating 200 calories a day less than you do right now could result in a weight loss of twenty pounds in a year!

making smarter choices and maximizing the benefits from the training you are doing.

Poor nutrition, on the other hand, is a guaranteed way to limit the end result of a great exercise program. In the extreme, it may cause you to end up with a broken-down physical machine.

3 Set a Goal— Change Your Life

Having a positive experience from your fitness helps drive health changes for life. The first step to doing this for any person, family, or couple is to choose an exercise you like to do. Then, using those forms of exercise that spark your interest, set fitness and health goals challenging enough to draw you into action, but realistic enough to be attainable over time.

Without a commitment to creating long-term lifestyle change, your immersion in the world of fitness will probably be temporary. There's always a surge of excitement in the beginning, fueled by the hope and vision of a healthier, leaner, and fitter you. That enthusiasm can drive people to look for quick results to support their immediate vision of change.

But fast beginnings cannot be sustained, plain and simple. When things naturally start to slow down, it can be frustrating . . . unless a solid, long-term vision has been put in place to keep you going.

Mark: According to Plan I had a conversation with a guy who said he is always sore when he works out. He started with the intention of working out five days a week for six weeks. The plan was three days of aerobic exercise and two days in the gym. He was consistent for two weeks, but then it declined to one day a week of aerobics and one day at the gym. That is just enough activity to make him sore every single time he goes out there. This is a formula that will most likely end in an aborted program.

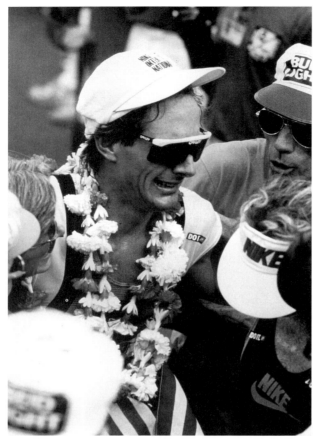

The emotion that comes from attaining a goal is unbelievable! In 1989 I finally won the Ironman on my seventh attempt. My entire family was there at the finish to celebrate with me.

Changes in your level of health and fitness, if gauged on the scale of your lifetime, actually occur pretty quickly. Over a few weeks or months, you will feel a major difference. Once you do, keep going to maintain it. Commit to a lifetime of health by working out a day at a time.

Make It Yours Creating a fitness plan that is enjoyable and effective is not difficult. What can be tough is getting past those personal blocks that exist somewhere inside you. All the knowledge in the world is like ether if a fear or bad habit keeps you from taking the first step.

Part of achieving physical fitness and health is finding a way to bolster your mental and emotional circuitry to match the task. It's about finding the courage to start and having the humility to stick with it. It sounds easy, but sometimes your self-image gets in the way.

Who are some of our most notable public figures? Supermodels and professional athletes. These very public images of physicality are unrealistic and can be motivationally damaging to both men and women. We tend to forget that their *job* is to be beautiful and/or fit—they work at it twenty-four hours a day.

Most women who resist exercising do it because of past negative experiences and an inability to meet standards that don't mesh with the reality of their bodies. Men's fears about working out are more related to feeling inadequate in a culture where the expectation that males will fit an athletic mold is so pervasive.

One of the best ways to get beyond the discrepancy between your body type and that of your superheroes is to take up an activity that you truly enjoy, not one that you are doing solely to change your body type. Then commit to a realistic six-week plan that you can stick to and use as your own personal template for transformation.

Mark: Getting in Shape One of the biggest fears that hold people back from working out is that they are not in shape. I go through that all the time. It hit me hardest after I quit racing. After I retired, I stopped working out for three months. I went from world-class athlete to couch potato overnight.

After two and a half months, I had put on maybe five pounds, which is not that significant. Two weeks later, I had gained another five pounds. The curve had been level for a long time, but it got very steep very quickly.

Uh-oh.

Ten pounds is not a big deal. But if I continued gaining that fast, it would *become* a big deal. It got my attention. At the same time, all my joints were stiff and my energy levels were slowly dropping—the opposite of what I thought would happen from just sitting around.

Finally, as reluctant as I was to work out as a normal guy instead of a professional athlete, I did it. The mirrors in the gym didn't lie. Nor did the scale at home or my darling wife, who was pinching much more than an inch around my midsection.

It took about three more months before I was back down to my normal weight. My body composition is still not, and never will be, quite what it was during my career. But that is no longer the goal.

Julie: In and Out of Shape When I stepped away from triathlons in 1991, it was a relief to abandon the grind of three workouts a day while juggling a travel and competition schedule. After ten years of being a professional triathlete, I loved the idea of not having to work out. But it was a fantasy I indulged with limited success. The truth, I found out, was that being in shape had become a way of life, not an occupation.

After the luxury of lying about for several weeks, the restlessness got to me. I started to look around for an athletic project. Suddenly, the idea of running a marathon caught hold. The run segment of the triathlon had always been my weakest link. I began to relish the idea of focusing on only one event and seeing if I could develop beyond my self-image as a "bad" runner. I renewed friendships with old running buddies, the men and women who had attempted to teach me to run as a triathlete. They offered a noncompetitive environment for me to train in. With their help, I returned to the world of fitness, this time focusing just on running a good marathon.

The year 1991 was a fun time to be a female runner. With the upcoming Olympic trials, American women had a specific goal to shoot for. Any woman running 2:45 or faster would be invited to participate in the Olympic trials the following winter.

I chose the Boston Marathon for my debut. It was a magical race for me. I never felt the punishing miles of downhill running the first half of the event. Nor did I notice the aches from climbing world-famous Heartbreak Hill near the end. My time of 2:47:17 placed me twentieth overall! My name was printed (in very fine print) in the results of sports pages across America. It was an incredible personal success.

I'd come close to my goal time at Boston, and I'd have eight months to shave another two and a half minutes off to grab an Olympic trials invitation. I'd found my focus for the rest of the year.

I ran the Twin Cities Marathon six months later. At 20 miles, I was right on target, but the toughest 6 miles loomed large ahead. I felt I couldn't keep up the pace and thought it would be wiser to bank the 20-mile effort and try another marathon before the end-of-the-year cutoff for the trials. I did run a December marathon, but it was a disaster. I'd have to wait another four years to enter the Olympic trials.

Even though I failed to reach my ultimate goal, running had changed my life—and my perspective. Fitness was now without a doubt an integral part of my life. I saw that I didn't have to let my past image of being a poor runner hold me back. I fully understood the importance of having a training support system, both from my running buddies and my family, who handed me the time I needed to work out.

I also learned that it's not always accomplishing the end goal that empowers you. I didn't make the Olympic trial standard. But I found the courage to pursue the dream, and doing that has changed my life forever.

Envision the Possibilities All successful people had a vision in place before they took that first step. Allowing that vision to change and evolve over time is the elastic that keeps it alive.

It's very important to develop your own vision, your own fitness goals. They serve as a magnet to draw you into action. Having clearly defined goals helps keep your energy and enthusiasm levels up when plateaus in progress try to derail you from consistency in training. Without them, it is easy to get lost in the mileage or daily weigh-ins and forget that there are bigger reasons you are out there every day.

Very few people will stick with a fitness program just because they "want to feel better." The needs of the workday, kids, and just about every other real-world obligation can easily sideline training that is done just to feel good. It sets you up to feel guilty—taking all that time and energy just so you can feel good!

Mark: Potential Potential, possibility, who you can be, what you can change—that's vision. It doesn't require knowing all the steps to get there. It only becomes a nightmare when you get stuck in the not-knowing and don't take the first action to fulfill your vision.

In the Beginning Start with a vision of what you want your life to be. Take some time, let your mind wander, use your imagination. Don't base your goals on someone else's vision. Find your own. Be honest, but don't be afraid to dream big. And don't try to do too many things at once. Start out with one overriding fitness goal. Phrase your goal as an "I will," not an "I want to." Then write it down, say it out loud, post it where you'll see it every day.

You may surprise yourself about what you really want. You may horrify yourself with how big your true goals are. Relax. Break your goal down into small steps, or secondary goals. Write these down, too, and then tackle the first one. If your goal is to lose thirty pounds, your first step will be to set up an exercise program. What do you need to do this? Think it through. Do you need to join a health club? Find a congenial walking group? Take a class? If your goal is to improve your swimming, you can find a coach, join a Masters swim group, go to swim camp. No matter how big or small your goal is, there's always a first step. Figure out what that is—and take it.

Make sure each step is measurable, something you can take pride in achieving. That can be the carrot that keeps your commitment going. Reward yourself for reaching each step toward your overall goal, and don't beat yourself up if it takes longer than you think it should. Stay positive, even if that means retraining your brain. Meditation and the use of mantras or affirmations can help.

Hunt out a support system that will be involved along the way and help keep you going when the lazy side wants to take over and alter your good intentions. If your partner already works out, hitch your wagon to his or hers until you develop goals of your own. If you are both just getting going, set your goals together, then provide a friendly support, making whatever allowances you must.

Mark: The Bottom Line I never competed in an Ironman where I could see myself winning during every moment of the event. Every single one had small eternities where I had to fall back on my bottom-line goal, which was just to finish. Doing that would at least honor all the people who had given their help to get me ready for the race. Without a doubt, my ultimate goal was to win, but my bottom-line goal was to cross the finish line. And it was having these different layers of goals that helped me to continue on when my legs were screaming at me to quit. Fortunately, more often than not my body did come around. But if my *only* goal had been to win, I would have certainly given up when it looked like it had slipped out of my reach.

Julie: Having a Goal It's not the actual goal that is important; it's having one that gets you heading in a positive direction. Create goals for *you*, ones that fit who you are and where you are starting from. A realistic goal for one person might be simply to open the door every Tuesday and walk around the block three times. It can be social if you do it with your family or with a friend. While walking, look around. Drink in those moments, notice the light, the movement of air around you, the smells. You can see some things you can't see when driving in a car or riding a bicycle. You won't hurt yourself if you actually look at a beautiful hawk that flies overhead. Learn to enjoy the achievement of your goal.

Even though it should be realistic, a goal should also stretch you some. For me, it's the stretch that sparks me to continually explore my own fitness. Going beyond your comfort zone can open up an incredible world that you would never experience if you always play it safe. I found this out in 1982, when I dreamed about doing the Ironman. At the time, I thought

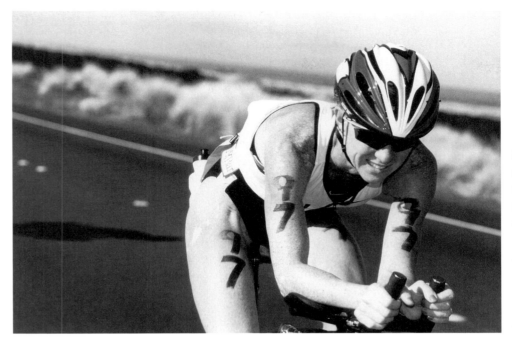

Because I did not complete the race during my last attempt at the Ironman, I felt that for closure's sake it was important to finish in Kona one more time. In 1997 Mark and I reversed roles: He watched the race as a commentator for NBC while I competed in it.

of *walking* as a major challenge. I didn't know what I was getting myself into; I just wanted to get ready for it and go. It was a huge stretch. But because I followed my dream, because I went for it even though it sounded unreasonable, a whole different perspective on what I could do opened up. In the end, it defined an entire sport—and me.

I put things in a competitive context when I set goals. Without something to push me, I would be content to go back to my fall-back workout forever. I would be happy just finding my lowest watermark of fitness instead of my highest. There has to be something big out there to make all the time and energy worth it.

Destination races are great way to set double payoff goals. Train for a marathon, but pick one in a city you have always wanted to see. The London Marathon—why not? Just going there would be the trip of a lifetime. And combining your goals is the heart and soul of a great lifestyle. There is nothing like racing the streets and seeing the people who live in a different locale coming out and supporting the event. You can gain a lifetime of memories in one day, even though the meat and potatoes of the experience are set in the day-to-day workouts that help get you there.

Clarify Your Goals Sit quietly by yourself and close your eyes, keeping yourself relaxed, yet alert. Now remember your ultimate goal and visualize it happening. See, feel, and experience all the sensations around the scene at the moment that you achieve the goal. Let the joy and satisfaction of that moment fill your heart. You have made your goal a reality, because in your mind's eye you have just seen it and in your heart you have felt it.

Now visualize the things you did in the week leading up to your success that allowed you to achieve that goal. Then look into the crystal ball of your mind and see what you did in the week before that. Keep working your way back to the present, noticing all the things you did along the way that enabled you to achieve your ultimate goal.

By working your way back to the present, you will have a much clearer picture of what is necessary to accomplish your goal than if you start by looking at today and asking what it will take to get from here to the finish line. Starting at the end and working backward is the same as someone giving you a car engine, having you disassemble it, then asking you to put it together. You saw what it looked like in its completed form and at every stage along the way.

Starting with today, on the other hand, and working forward is like someone giving you all the pieces of a car engine and asking you to put it together without ever having the advantage of seeing what it looked like in one piece. Approaching your goals this way is like someone dumping shoes, goggles, a bike, and a bunch of nutritional supplements on your doorstep and telling you to take that stuff and go complete an Ironman. It's much easier the other way around!

Julie: Self-Motivation

Self-motivation is overrated. It has a very short shelf life—you go through your bag of tricks, then you're stuck. Use your friends (other people are much better motivators than you are) and training partners (who don't have to be your friends). A coach or training partner takes you to the next consistent level. How many people have a membership to a gym and don't go? There's a difference between intention and motivation.

Make a Start

How do you set goals that integrate fitness into your life? First, you have to make fitness a priority. It won't happen on its own. Every time you have a choice to fit in a workout or blow it off, try opting for the one that adds to fitness, not the one that puts it off for another day. Don't think about it. Just do it.

Having the time to work out and doing something with that time are two very different things. It's easy to *think* about how you are going to work out, or what activity you are *planning* to do when the time presents itself. In moderate amounts, thinking and planning are important steps in the big picture of putting a smart training program together. But too much thinking and planning can eat up more energy than actually getting out there and exercising. Visualizing a 10-mile run while sitting in front of the computer screen just won't go very far in reducing the waistline and increasing lean muscle mass. It takes putting on the shoes, going out the door, and taking the first step in what hopefully will become a lifetime of journeys along your path of fitness.

Mark: Memorable Moments

If I think about the most memorable moments in my life, none of them happened when I was lounging in a chair somewhere. They all happen out there past the edge of my current level of comfort. Afterward, I can spend time in the easy chair absorbing that effort, race, or hard workout. That's when the pleasure can balance pushing my mind and body to new heights.

There Are No Excuses

Remember, your life changes, the situation changes, and so should your goals. If the absolute dream goal is the only way you will be happy at the end of the line, you have almost nixed any chance of achieving it. There are just too many moments when that goal may seem out of reach, moments that instantaneously become pivotal points where doubt can blow your resolve to continue into a million useless pieces. There may also come a time when that goal doesn't seem worth the effort. It's just not as important to you anymore. So sit down and think about what *is* important, and refocus yourself on a new or refined or expanded goal.

Some days, it is easy to see your goal happening. Other days, it seems like an impossibility. This will happen over and over along the path you journey from the start to the realization of your goal. It's normal. It happens in races. It happens in life. There is never a race where you will visualize reaching your goal during every moment of the event. There are always periods where the challenge of the day becomes greater than your ability to see your goal as a real possibility. It's the same for losing weight, gaining strength, raising your kids, sustaining your marriage, hitting your targets at work.

This is when having several levels of goals will help. Let's say that your ultimate goal is to finish in the top 100 at the Ironman. Unfortunately, at the beginning of the run you find yourself positioned somewhere around five hundredth. Your ultimate goal may seem like an absurdly unachievable fantasy at that moment. If finishing in the top 100 was your only goal, it would be very easy to give up at that

I f you can't come up with an intriguing goal on your own, here are a few to chew on. And remember, no matter what your goal, it takes about six weeks to develop a new pattern of behavior, a positive habit of health. It also takes about six weeks of training to start to see significant changes in your fitness level.

• Enter a 5K walk for charity, or a 10K, a half marathon, a triathlon—an event that stretches you past your current level of fitness. Make sure it's at least three months away. Then train for it. This is a measurable goal with a deadline—the best kind. Organize smaller goals to keep you on track toward the larger fitness goal. There is nothing like it when you cross the finish line after months of getting ready.

• Take the next six months to work up to running forty-five minutes—again, a measurable goal with a deadline. Start out by measuring how long you can run. Then set your first goal to double that time, always keeping the ultimate goal in mind. If you can run for fifteen minutes now, you need to be able to run for thirty minutes in three months to make it to forty-five minutes in six months. Do the math, then do the work.

• Prepare for all-women's sporting events like the Danskin all-women triathlons. You don't have to worry about body image in that kind of environment, and the distances are short enough to be doable with six to nine weeks of working out consistently.

• Work out (don't diet) until you are a size smaller in your favorite clothes. A measurable goal, but a deadline would give it more urgency.

• Earn the calories for a great meal. Keep track of the calories you burn working out and spend them on a special evening. If you're consistent, you can order it all, from soup to nuts, appetizer to dessert. If you're smart, you'll go dancing afterward and start filling your calorie account back up.

• Plan a physical outing with your mate a month from now. Set a date. Then get fit enough to enjoy rather than dread it. This has a deadline but isn't very measurable. Still, making physical activities part of your relationship is an excellent lifestyle goal.

• Complete a strength training program in preparation for your favorite sport that you only get to do a handful of times each year, like skiing or mountain climbing. Ski season starts December 1; three months of regular weight training and in-line skate workouts should have you ready.

• Learn a new sport: golf, tennis, surfing, kayaking. Have you ever used a crampon? A snowboard? Whatever you choose, just do it because it excites you. To make this measurable and give it a deadline, join a class or find an instructor and take lessons. If you pay for it in advance, you're more likely to be there on time and prepared to learn.

---

point or just slog through the final leg of the race.

But what if one of your secondary goals was to finish in under fourteen hours? By your estimation at the start of the marathon, let's say you figure out that, if you could come up with a fairly solid marathon, you would probably finish around 13:30. Suddenly, you don't feel like the day is a total waste. In fact, you start to become absorbed in making that under-fourteen-hour cutoff, temporarily forgetting about the top 100 mark.

Now the possibility of something amazing is set in motion. You are placing yourself squarely in position to achieve a goal you set for yourself. You have also freed up your attachment to having to attain the entire original goal to get any satisfaction out of the race. You haven't given up on the day—or on yourself.

Suddenly, you are coming up on the turn-around point of the marathon and it is obvious that you have passed quite a few competitors in the first half of the run. It is becoming apparent that not only are you going to go well under fourteen hours for the day, but you have a chance to finish in the top 200! It's not your ultimate goal, but it is closer.

More miles go by, and you are on a roll. By 20 miles, you come to the realization that it doesn't matter where you finish. What is most important is to just give it everything you have. You cross the line, look up and see number 97 on the clock. You did it. Top 100! And it only happened because your stepping-stone goals kept you going when the ultimate one looked impossible.

These secondary goals are not excuses to do less than your best. They are steps *toward* being your best—and each step is significant, something to be proud of, something that leads you toward the top.

Tell Your Partner What You Are Up To Give your partner a menu of goals you have for yourself. You have relationship goals, work goals; now incorporate your fitness goals into the picture. Then work out the dynamics. Once you tell another person what your goals are, every time you start to deviate, you have to look him in the face. Your partner is the greatest truth serum there is. When you let someone else know what you are trying to accomplish, he can help you keep your focus. Then you can work together to help carve out the space and the time you need to do the work to reach your goals.

Be as truthful as you can. If you tell your partner that you just want to get a little fitter when your real goal is to win the Eco-Challenge, you might end up in divorce court. He thinks you want to go to the gym one or two days a week, and he adjusts for that. Meanwhile, you are training hours on end and need him to make major adjustments. Be honest. If he knows your real goal, it might become a joint project, and he can really help you realize it.

Mark: A Partnership Hopefully, both members of the partnership will have athletic goals. Julie and I have naturally different preferences as to when our bodies work best. She is best very early in the morning. I need a little time to get rolling. Neither of us is very good late in the day, but both of us will take working out late in the day over no workout at all. The more

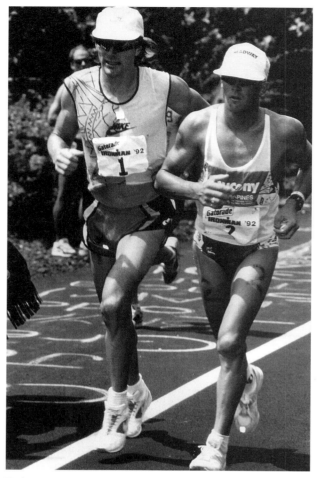

To become the best competitor you can be, you need more than your friends and family: You need someone to share the race with you. In 1992 it was Australian star Greg Welch who pushed me early (above) and then Cristian Bustos of Chile who made my life miserable late in the marathon. I waited for Cristian at the finish and we greeted the crowd together (right).

you understand about each other's preferences and can follow that genetic blueprint, the better off you'll be.

Julie: I Just Feel Better It's taken me a long time to understand that I feel better when I work out. The best time for me to do it is in the morning. It seems to set my metabolic and energy levels for the day.

Adopt a Long-Term Perspective After settling into the basics of your fitness program, you might find yourself ready to attempt a more

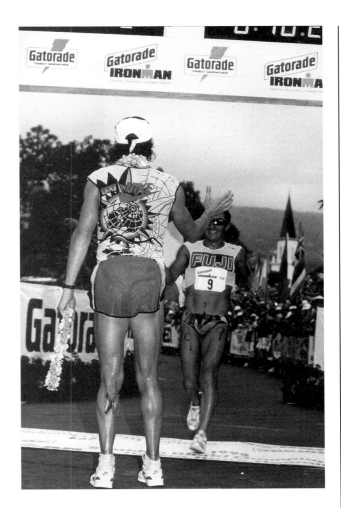

winter when the cold and bad weather can be stumbling blocks to a training program. I always start out with good intentions, but I can slide unless I have a goal. It also helps me get through the holiday eating and celebrating patterns that I can slide into. If you have to get up on Sunday for a big workout, you tend to employ more moderation.

I'm not talking about being militant with my program. It's more about just keeping at least some of my focus on it. Then I can start the New Year with five pounds to get rid of instead of ten pounds. It makes the job doable instead of overwhelming.

Mark: Trade-Offs
When you have a family, you will have to make trade-offs. Since Mats arrived—he is five now—Julie and I have taken turns in the workout department. The first two years of Mats's life, the workout focus was definitely on me, partly because I was still racing and that was how we made our living. Julie took care of the baby and used what little time was left over for her own fitness. For the last couple of years, Julie has worked out more.

On a day-to-day basis, our arrangement may not look balanced. But we don't look at fitness on a day-to-day basis for success or failure. We look at it over a broad expanse of time. You achieve balance in your various fitness programs with your partner over the long haul.

The Practical Guide
Are you totally and completely satisfied with your fitness right now? If you are, congratulations. If not, here is a guide to help up the chance of success and fulfillment from the goals that might be eluding you.

- **Up the volume and/or frequency.** Add additional workout volume in increments of fifteen to thirty minutes per week to your total weekly workout time. Up the volume for two weeks, then hold steady for one. Repeat this three-week cycle until you see the results you are after.

- **Commit to a balanced diet of fitness.** This means every week doing two strength workouts, at least three and a half hours of aerobic work-

challenging regimen. A bigger challenge will probably require more of your time—which might also equate to less time for everyone else in your household. It happens all the time. There is usually one member of any couple who is more enthusiastic. The other can feel frustration: "My boyfriend works out all the time. Now he runs with buddies or he's at the pool and he is tired at night. When will this ever end?"

Try to involve your partner with your new goals. Maybe you want to run a marathon. Ask your partner to run with you—or at least to start your run with you. While you run, he or she can ride the bike, carrying enough water for both of you. It becomes a mutual effort to meet on different grounds.

Julie: Good Intentions
Setting a springtime goal is one of the most important things I do, because it keeps me focused throughout the

Spice Up Your Program

Maybe the program is working but it's starting to feel a little stale. Here are a few goals to shoot for that can spice it up.

• Explore a new frontier to keep from getting stale. If the 10K was good, how about a half marathon or a triathlon?

• Tired of a road bike? There's a whole new world out there on the trails. Get a mountain bike and go see.

• Is the gym feeling like a worn-out shoe? See what's happening outside the walls and the beat of the dance music. It may require more bundling up in the winter, or doing it with a friend to get you out of bed early. But if it keeps the routine from becoming routine, it's worth it.

• Missing your family on those solo training programs? End up at a park, a stream, the top of a mountain—wherever you think they would enjoy meeting you and having some family time. Just say no to the television. Any show will look even better after your workout is done and you are free to watch it on the video.

• Have you hit a plateau? Every program has them, those points where fitness is good, but the next level seems elusive. Try this: One week every month, up your normal workout volume by 25 percent to 30 percent. The other weeks, simply keep things as they are. You should notice a significant improvement from doing this even once.

• Looking for a real test? Try upping your weekly workout volume by 25 percent to 30 percent from your current level every other week for six weeks. The alternate weeks, stay at your current level. Be cautious of possible overuse injuries, though. If you feel them coming, back off. If not, just keep going. This type of stress-and-recovery cycle in training is one of the secrets of champions. Upping the ante in training then recovering from it makes for huge leaps in fitness.

outs, and incorporating flexibility work—especially if you feel some nagging pain or soreness from workouts.

• **Pick a race goal.** Estimate the approximate amount of time it will take you to finish your event. Then make sure one of your workout days each week has a total workout time equivalent to 75 percent to 100 percent of the time it will take you to finish the race. If your goal is a 10K and you guess it will take you forty minutes to complete it, have one workout each week that is about forty minutes long. For long endurance events, choose the lower end of the scale. For example, an estimated four-hour marathon could be serviced with a sampling of three-hour runs in the weeks leading up to it.

Integrate Fitness into Your Life To increase your chances of earning that fitness pot of gold, take a look at some of the other areas of life that affect your fitness and incorporate them into a solution that will lead to your goal.

Diet. Are you getting enough protein, essential fats, and complex carbohydrates? If not, make the changes necessary to bring it back into balance. Do you slug down too much refined sugar? Slow the flow. How's the portion size? Working out thirty to forty minutes a day does not give you a license to pig out like a linebacker.

Rest. Without enough of it, your body cannot absorb the benefits of working out. Sometimes you will get stronger by skipping that extra run and sleeping in to help regenerate your tissues and the internal batteries.

Stress. Have you had too much lately? If so, do whatever it takes to reduce it. If the job isn't going to go away, go away from the job. This can be as complicated as taking a big vacation. It can be as simple as parking your body under an old tree and watching the sunset, breathing in the colors, and giving your mind and your heart something other than sales reports to absorb.

Reality and Fantasy. We all have our dream goals: lose fifty pounds, run a marathon, hike the Pacific Crest Trail. But the training program you design and are living may be only good enough to present the illusion that you are getting ready for the goal. Go to the end of the line, see the goal, work back, and ask yourself if you are really headed in the right direction. Do this every so often. Call it a reality check.

Just Keep Going The one stumbling block to fulfilling any goal is the amount of time it takes to get there. Setting a goal can take some time and some real introspection. Developing the logistics for a plan of action that will help you realize that goal might take an evening or two talking it over with your family and training partners. Seeing the dream result in your life could take two years.

Most people, unfortunately, refuse to wait it out. We live in a society where everything comes fast. Can you e-mail me that document right now? Can you fax me fitness in five minutes? Can you scan me that new body? Can you FedEx me the ability to win a race? *I need it now!*

The Right Focus Most people think focus is a steely resolve that never wavers. They imagine a champion as someone who can hold that picture every moment of every step along the road to achieving excellence. It sounds superhuman.

Focus is often associated with athletics, and especially with endurance events that seem to define going beyond the normal standards of human possibility. It requires focus to keep going when the difficulty of a race gets extreme. Yet focus is even more important over the long-term training needed to do a race like the Ironman.

No one is strong enough to hold his or her focus on a goal without letting it go periodically along the way. No one has the capacity to keep a focus at its highest level for months on end. So you're human. Your environment, circumstances, and energy levels alternate between making it easy to be focused on your final goal and making it virtually impossible.

Long-term focus requires modifying the moment-to-moment focus to match the dynamics of life. Try to keep your goal in sight

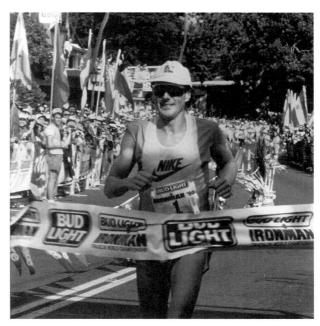

Nothing feels better than breaking a finish line tape.

and keep taking the steps to get there. Then, when you are tired or bored, let it go. It will come back. Just keep going forward, keep going through the motions. Over the long term, you don't have to be locked into a superhumanly narrow focus. Save that stuff for the race.

Mark: Completion Taking something all the way to completion, no matter what—that's an empowering experience. It brings new strength, knowledge, and understanding that fulfills you on a much different and often deeper level than even winning does.

In my third Hawaii Ironman, I was going for the win. It was 1984. I had raced the event twice before. The first time, I didn't finish because my derailleur, the transmission of my bike, broke partway through the bike ride and I couldn't shift gears. The second time, I finished third with an effort that felt like I gave about 80 percent of what I could. This time, I was ready to put it all on the line, fully expecting that it would lead to victory.

Starting the run, I was leading the field. My fiercest competitor was Dave Scott, who came into that race a two-time Ironman champion. He was twelve minutes behind me, too far back to be a threat. At 10K into the marathon, I

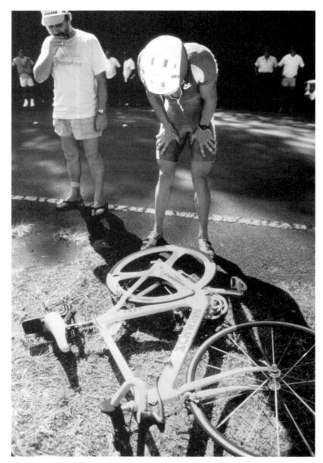

I had a lot of bad luck competing on the Kona Coast of Hawaii. In 1988 I had two flat tires and ended up in fifth place.

knew I would win. At 20K, I had slowed to a jog. At about 30K, I was walking—and being passed by not only Dave Scott, but also a host of others.

The final 10 miles were a supreme test. I struggled, walking twenty steps, then jogging as many as I could. I was working at about 20 percent of what my maximum capacity was on a good day—but I was squeezing 100 percent out of that 20 percent situation. I finished fifth that year. Dave Scott won. I didn't. But I could hold my head high because I had given all I could.

Perhaps the most difficult thing to do is to live the truth of what you are asking for in your life. When you throw yourself into something that could have a very fulfilling payoff, there is almost always a challenge. To go beyond that challenge, you have to face a level of truth about yourself that you're either afraid to face or were unaware of.

In 1984, I thought I could win. The reality was that I arrived at the race underprepared and overanxious. By surrendering to that truth and going on anyway, I found a strength and patience about myself that I never knew existed. I was able to use it many years later on the flip side of my career, when I finally won the Ironman.

Julie: Failure Throughout my career, there was a pattern of incompletion that began at the Ironman in 1985 and continued in 1989 and 1990. I dropped out of all three of those events well before crossing the finish line. This pattern emerged again later in my marathons. These races came back to haunt me. As the years went by, all my second-guessing solidified into regret. In the heat of the moment, my decisions to drop out were absolutely justified. I tried to be kind to myself and leave those decisions out on the lava fields where they belonged—away from the objective reality of a comfortable condo the day after the race.

However, once I was inducted into the Ironman Hall of Fame in 1993, the little voice in my head started to become louder. I knew one day I would have to settle the score. I owed it to myself to feel a sense of completion about my career in Kona, especially since my name would be brought up with each new annual induction into the Hall of Fame. While watching the race in 1996, it became completely clear I would be back the following year to finish up what I'd started. I was ready to reclaim my right to stand tall in Kona and be counted as an Ironman.

Had I known that it would take me six years to undo the damage to my psyche caused by dropping out of the Ironman in Hawaii, I never would have dropped out. I'd have found a way to get to the finish and saved myself from the slow, insidious stalking of failure. Now I had a chance to redo history, and I wasn't going to waste a minute of it.

The year 1997 was the most stress-free year

of training I can ever remember. The workouts flowed along like clockwork. I can count on one hand the days when it was hard to get out the door. I was completely focused and motivated. In hindsight, I knew my ego had gotten the better of me in Kona, where it hadn't been good enough just to finish. I felt I had to finish top 10, and once I'd been passed for tenth, I was a failure. This time, I knew my ego was the enemy and I was going to create limitless opportunities for success upon my return to Kona.

I went to Australia in April to do a tune-up Ironman. I needed a chance to be a rookie in semi-obscurity. The Aussie event was low-key and a beautiful place to hang out for a week. All my focus and hard training paid off, and my race far exceeded my expectations. I won my age group, thirty-five to forty, and was seventh woman overall. I distinctly remember my first thought, that this race was too good, I should quit now. But my demons resided in Kona and our date in October was long overdue.

I had three goals for myself before I stepped off the plane in Kona for the 1997 Ironman. The first was just get to the finish, no strings attached and no egos allowed. The second was to be willing to give to the race rather than take from it. And the third was to smile as I crossed the line.

My final Ironman experience was just as challenging as I feared. I needed every bit of training and experience to get me to the finish line. When the demons called my name and found me walking in the lava fields at mile 18 of the marathon, I smiled at them and they grew quiet. By mile 20, I was running again and I knew that now my race was with the sun to see if I could finish before it set. I won. I gave myself every opportunity to win my battle with Kona and my October demons, and I won. I was second in my age group, but that distinction pales in comparison to the war I waged in my head.

Later that night, Mark and I returned to the finish-line celebration to welcome home the last finishers. For several hours, I cheered for my fellow Ironman competitors, who won their personal battles with Kona and stepped across the line into a very exclusive club. I stood tall as I heralded their arrival and knew that, in this new version of my Ironman story, I had no regrets and no wasted moments.

Mark: Fulfillment Completing a goal that took time, work, and dedication to accomplish—there's nothing more fulfilling. But more subtle than that is simply feeling as though there is a balance between my workouts, family, work, activity, and quiet, between physical, emotional, intellectual, and spiritual strengths. Being able to focus on each step along the way can be as satisfying as the step that takes me to a win at the Ironman, because both are just affirmations that I am out there living my life to the fullest.

4 The Energy Pie—Creating the Time

Now you have some definable fitness goals. That part was easy. In the upcoming chapters, the mechanics of how to accomplish those goals are spelled out. That, too, will be easy. The essentials of good training follow your nature as a human being. It just makes sense.

The most difficult part of accomplishing anything you set out to do is finding the time and energy for it. This takes pieces of what you can think of as an Energy Pie. Everyone has one. It's where the energy for your life gets served from on a daily basis. A huge slice is eaten up by your job. Another is reserved for your family. Hopefully, by the time the workout rolls around, there is still something left on the pie plate.

A Recipe for Life Let's look at the two main ingredients in the Energy Pie: time and energy. Giving a piece to one area of your life makes it unavailable for another. Serving up twelve hours of time and energy from your daily pie to work means that time and energy is not available for family, workouts, or the unexpected things that crop up here and there, like traffic jams and drop-in visitors. It becomes a daily balancing act to find a way to slice and serve without running out of pieces toward the end of the day. This job can make the Ironman look like a walk in the park.

Here is one solution: It's called *prioritizing*. It's a simple formula. The things you think are most important get served first, while those low on the list may find the energy pie empty when it's their turn. By moving fitness up on the priority list, you can make sure you have enough time and energy available for training.

The biggest challenge here is the ever-changing nature of life. The way you split up the Energy Pie today may look nothing like what it will a year from now. Our lives are always evolving.

Mark: Life Changes A friend of mine couldn't figure out why his workouts were going backward. Every time out the door, he was running slower and feeling worse than the day before. Over lunch one day, I asked him what had changed in his life.

In the previous six months he had gotten married and bought a house, and he and his wife had their first child. He had gone from a single, carefree workoutaholic to a responsible adult with a house and a family with little time to adjust emotionally or physically. In other words, he had doubled the number of areas in his life that needed pieces of his pie without expanding the size of the actual pie itself. While the amount of time and energy expended for work had stayed the same, he had less time and energy available for sleep, for working out, for just goofing off.

Once he could step back and actually look at his Energy Pie, it was pretty obvious that he had to totally rethink his priorities and figure out how to make everything work.

Finding the Time Often the Energy Pie gets divvied up long before any of it gets put aside for fitness. This is a reality. Who wants to get up at some ridiculously early hour to work out before heading into the office? Who has the energy left at the end of the day to pack in thirty painful minutes of exercise?

Fitness is no longer a byproduct of living. You have to *make* it happen. Exercise requires physical energy to accomplish—and often a big dose of mental energy just to get out the door. Both of these elements take hefty slices out of the Energy Pie. Sometimes just the thought of adding a workout on to the other commitments in your life can be enough to activate the internal overload button.

So where can you find the time? How can you create the energy?

At first glance, it may look as if there is a finite amount of energy and time to split up. You need ten to twelve hours of energy and time for work and the commute in both directions. Another chunk has to be carved out to fulfill all the daily household and family commitments. Then, even the most sleep-deprived human spends some time in the sack. Where can you possibly find another thirty minutes or hour of that time pie to work out?

Scheduling: The Anatomy of a Day
Here is a realistic model of a twenty-four-hour period in the average adult American's day:

The alarm goes off at six A.M. It takes forty-five minutes to get to work with the traffic. You have to be at your desk at eight A.M., but everyone shows up ten to fifteen minutes early at your company. So you rush through a shower, scan the paper while you grab some toast and coffee, and by seven A.M. it's out the door.

You work all morning, then have one hour for lunch. You take only from twelve-thirty to one P.M., however, because it's expected. In that half hour, you only have time for a fast-food fix and more coffee, hurrying all the time.

You are supposed to get off by five P.M., but there are projects that need to get done and people you need to talk to in different time zones. So you don't get out of the office until six-thirty at best. Most days it's seven.

You get home pretty close to eight P.M., unless you have to stop by the market or the bank first—and finally it's time for you. Forget a workout. You're starving, exhausted, and, well, tomorrow's another day. So you eat something that resembles dinner from eight-thirty to nine P.M. By the time the dishes are cleaned up, it's nine-thirty.

By then the day is D-O-N-E and so are you. The mind and body need some time to wind down. You look at mail, read magazines, and, the next thing you know, it's eleven P.M. If you don't get to bed now, tomorrow is going to be a nightmare. Eleven P.M. to six A.M. is the buffer between today and tomorrow. If you're lucky, your mind won't try to solve the world's problems tonight and you will get some sleep.

And you don't even have kids yet.

Planning Makes a Difference Where is this person going to find the time to work out? Here are ten suggestions for this situation that probably mirror the reality many Americans live in.

1. Get up just a little bit earlier. Skip the shower, climb in the car, and drive to the health club wearing your workout clothes. Bring your business clothes organized on a hanger. By getting your training in before work, it's done and your mind is free to focus on the rest of the day. Energy is created with that freedom. Time is created because you miss rush-hour traffic, and your mind and body are humming, so you're productive from the moment you enter your office. The Energy Pie is working for you instead of against you.

2. You don't like getting up early? What are you doing for lunch? Conduct that business conversation in running shoes instead of over a glob of chicken Caesar salad. Get your boss to join you for a noon indoor cycling class at the club. Start a lunchtime walking group. (There's strength in numbers.) This is a whole hour of your Energy Pie.

3. Pack your workout clothes in the gym bag and keep them in the trunk of the car. Then you can do a workout on your way home, before collapsing into the easy chair. Take that run in the park before Junior asks you to help with homework that not even you can figure out. The bottom line here is that once you get home at the end of the day, the chance of getting out again is slim. So take the extra time before you head for home. Do a workout, and create more energy by transforming leftover, stagnant, sitting-in-the-office-chair energy into clean, oxygenated, workout-generated alive energy.

4. Meet your mate for a postwork, predinner swim. It'll get the juices flowing, and it always helps to have support. Your Energy Pie will be a little smaller in terms of time, but significantly bigger in terms of energy.

5. You have a family that needs and wants you around and who would strangle you if you didn't come straight home from work? Get some exercise equipment for the house. Put a treadmill in the garage or family room. You can work out at home, and the family knows you are at least within shouting distance. Get some free weights, a workout bench, and a floor mat. Use these to create your own circuit workout setup and invite the whole family to participate.

6. Give up some of your sacred television time and replace it with a workout. The average American watches about thirty hours of TV a week. Even a professional athlete would be hard-pressed to work out thirty hours in a week.

7. Do the workouts that require the most time on the days you have the time to do them. Stressing to fit in a two-hour workout on the bike during a one-hour lunch break defeats one of the benefits of exercise, which is stress reduction.

8. Cut back on work. Yes, just do it. Those reports, e-mails, faxes, projects, and briefs will still be there when you get back from your workout. And chances are you will be more efficient with better health and more energy than the slug next to you who wouldn't dream of skipping out early to meet people for a bike ride.

9. Meet your husband or wife, friend, or family member for a workout. Just knowing they will be waiting helps create the energy and motivation that may not exist when you are solo.

10. Use unexpected free time. Unexpected things get in the way of a workout, evaporate time, or drain your energy. But what happens when a slot of time suddenly opens up? Do you fill it with more work, just sit and vegetate, or head out for a quick jog? Do you burn up the time chatting with someone or invite them to sneak away for a walk? Do you go buy that dress you've been eyeing or fit in the workout that will make you feel better than any piece of clothing ever could?

Mark: Nooners I belong to a health club in La Jolla, California. It's right in the middle of downtown. We have several large groups of business people who come in at lunchtime to do their workouts. They just make the time and do it, bringing gym clothes with them to work. Lunch gets eaten on the fly a lot of times, but the positives are worth it. They don't have to get up earlier or get home late. The camaraderie and support of knowing there is going to be a group there every day to connect with is tremendous. But perhaps the most important plus for the nooners is that it doesn't take time away from their families.

All It Takes Research says twenty minutes of aerobic activity three to five times a week is enough for health. That is the magic number. That level of exercise significantly reduces your risk of heart attack and heart disease. Anything over that has no statistically discernible benefit.

But there is a whole exciting world waiting beyond the minimum. There is a *huge* difference between twenty minutes a day, three times a week, and thirty to forty minutes a day, five to six days a week. There is a whole other level of what exercise can do for you beyond simply preventing a life-threatening disease.

With improved fitness, strength, and health comes an ability to deal with a lot more challenges in life. You create more energy in your body and use it in any form—physical or intellectual. You are plugged into the socket and the switch is on. You have taken that Energy Pie and souped it up, given it revitalized ingredients. Your energy has a stronger flavor. Working extra at the desk isn't such a big drain on your system. Cleaning out that dirty garage is an adventure instead of something that makes your back sore. Keeping up with the kids becomes a joy instead of a chore.

Two More Ingredients Part of the Energy Pie recipe involves two more words: *pleasure* and *pain*. Pleasure is the seasoning in your life. Simply put, there have to be positive feelings or pleasure from the things you do. If not, there is little chance you can sustain those activities over time, no matter how good they are for you.

The dilemma in the world of exercise is that not all bodies are created equal, so there is no one exercise that will keep everyone happy. Some people are addicted to the positive feeling they get from running. Others hate it. Swimming can be regenerative. It can also be the most foreign, unsatisfying sport ever if you are not comfortable in the water. There *is* an activity your body is made for, however. You just have to find it. Then you'll exercise because you love it, and your satisfaction will skyrocket.

Julie: Addiction and Priorities Addiction and priorities can get confused. If you are in a relationship with someone who doesn't exercise, he or she may view your workouts as a physical addiction. But the goal is to become a person in balance.

Mark: Addicted to Exercise An addiction is something that has power over you, something you can't keep from being drawn to. This doesn't necessarily mean that it is bad. Being addicted to alcohol is probably not good for anyone. Being addicted to exercise becomes a negative only when it throws the big picture of your life out of balance. I may have looked addicted to winning during my career, and there were certainly periods when my dedication to racing was not balanced. But then, nothing great comes out of mediocre efforts.

A New Perspective Serving up the Energy Pie with a new viewpoint, or new priorities, redistributes your time and energy so there is enough to go around to the things that *are* important, instead of being eaten up by those things that *seem* so pressing in the no-workout reality.

Leave the old images of your time and Energy Pies behind and create new ones. If it always seems as if there is no time available for working out, slice the pie up differently. Take a slice from somewhere else and designate it for your workout. If you don't feel there is enough energy left at the end of the day to move your body, pick a time when you are more likely to find some extra energy and plan to work out then.

Believe it or not, if you carve out the time for a workout, the world will not collapse.

Once you get into an exercise routine, the pie gets bigger. Working out in the right way creates more energy in your life. Eating smart does the same. So does becoming physically stronger. Balancing physical movement, mental activity, and quiet time to regenerate your body and spirit makes the Energy Pie *huge.* By doing this, you will not only transform your body; you might transform yourself from a bit of a stressed-out grump into somebody who is happier and nicer to be around.

Combining Your Time One of the best ways to get more out of your Energy Pie is to do two things at once—making one slice of the pie go twice as far. Combine family time with workout time. We've always included Mats in our healthy lifestyle. Make social hour workout hour. Plug in to friends who want to be active and fit. Replace a dinner date with a workout. It's motivating, it's healthy, and no one has to leave a tip.

Mark: Active Play We've always had active play in the park and the ocean. The best part is that Mats is developing patterns for a healthy lifestyle while he gets time with his parents.

As Mats gets older, there are so many things that we like to do together that are physical. We recently took a vacation with friends to Hawaii. We spent two days on long hikes into the mountains. Mats, at five years old, kept up with us. I hope in twenty years we will be able to keep up with him.

A lot of our friends are having children later in life. Seeing forty-year-olds with newborns is not uncommon. We are not a generation that can rely on the natural health that comes with youth to see us through with our children. It has to be a choice.

I like having that as a choice—a healthy lifestyle. The small sacrifice of time that I spend working out when I am away from my family is more than balanced out by the type of life we can live.

Julie: Birthday Run For Mats's fifth birthday, we decided it was time for a big party. There is nothing more intimidating to me than the thought of entertaining a group of small children. I tried to think of something that would keep them busy and burn up some excess energy.

We came up with the Mats Allen Birthday Fun Run. It started at our house with a tape strung across the street, then wound down to the neighborhood school half a mile away. The finish took them around the school grounds, and they all got a medal. It gave the kids a chance to run around and to feel a sense of accomplishment at the same time. They still got the cake and pizza, but, hopefully, they also got a taste of a healthy lifestyle too.

Mats: Birthday Fun My birthday party was fun. I could have run the whole time, kept running and running. If I had to choose again, I would pick an exercising party. I loooooooved it.

Mark: The Energy Pie in Action After I won my fifth Ironman Triathlon title in 1993, I needed to take a break from racing the Ironman. I took 1994 off to recharge my batteries. But when I came back in 1995, the rules of the game had changed. The whole world was racing at a faster speed than I had seen before. Being away from serious training and racing was great psychologically, but I really started to question if I could ever get back to the level of the rest of the athletes.

As the number of training days before the 1995 Ironman started to dwindle, I knew I had to take a serious look at my Energy Pie. I was a father now, and that required quality time I had a problem providing because I was so tired from the intensity of the Ironman training. I was working out as much as eight hours a day and sleeping at least ten. I was always tired and never felt quite recovered before the next day of training.

Julie and I decided the goal was no longer to win, but to make sure that, when I crossed the finish line in October, as a family we knew we had done everything possible to get me ready.

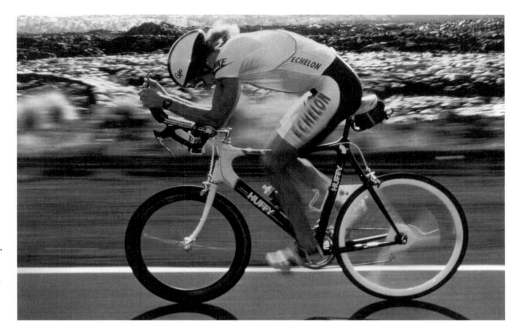

I have the ability to get inside myself and tune out the rest of the world. That skill came in handy while bicycling 112 mind-numbing miles through Hawaii's lava fields.

We wanted no regrets. The solution was for Mats and Julie to go back to our winter home in San Diego early and leave me in Boulder, Colorado, for the final four hard weeks of training, where I would hopefully build up the fitness I needed.

My job was to train without any distractions. It was a supreme sacrifice for our family, but it was necessary if I was going to be competitive with a field of tough competitors who were ten to fifteen years younger than I. By race morning, I would be thirty-seven years old. If I could win, I would become the oldest champion the race has ever seen. If I didn't, few would question why.

But the solution to my Ironman quest was only half answered by temporarily cutting family out of my Energy Pie. At thirty-seven, I could no longer outtrain the other athletes. My Energy Pie was smaller than theirs. If I was going to pull it off, I needed not only to train my body, I also had to become stronger at the core of my being. I needed to strengthen my heart and spirit.

So, before that final push of training in Boulder, the time that would test the limit of my "old guy" energy reserves, I did something that was totally contrary to conventional training wisdom. I took a week off from training—*completely* off. I went to a retreat in Alaska and joined the man who is my spiritual teacher, Brant Secunda.

Brant has been a shaman, healer, and ceremonial leader in the Huichol Indian tradition for over twenty years. Like most shamanic traditions, this one uses the power of nature to bring healing, balance, strength, and joy to people. I had spent many powerful times learning from Brant since I'd first met him in 1990. He had shared many exercises and led very traditional ceremonies to help strengthen who I am and to help me understand my own life through a direct connection with the spirit of nature.

But this time it was different. I needed more. I hadn't beaten any of my top competitors in over two years, and my prospects for the Ironman weren't looking good. If ever I needed Brant's help to expand my Energy Pie, to expand the realm of possibility, this was it.

For nine days, I surrounded myself with the power of Alaska, consciously nurturing my own natural strengths. With Brant's help, by the time I started my final push in Boulder, it felt as though my Energy Pie was back up to the size of a twenty-year-old's. Then the final touch, after eight intense weeks of endurance training, came on my way to Hawaii. I visited

Brant one last time before the race. That was what brought my energy back to world-class levels!

It was time to race. It didn't take long to see where the challenge would come from. Early in the 112-mile bike ride at the Ironman, a twenty-four-year-old German by the name of Thomas Hellriegel went by me like I was standing still. I thought, "The guy has never done this race before. How much time can he put on me?"

The kid put thirteen minutes on me during the bike ride. In the bike-to-run transition area, I knew I needed to run thirty seconds faster than he did—every single mile for 26.2 miles—if I wanted to catch him by the finish line. That was overwhelming.

I couldn't come anywhere close to visualizing a win at that moment. I wanted to give up and call it a career. But this was my last trip to Kona for the Ironman, so I couldn't quit. I remembered the sacrifice my family had made. That gave me immense strength. I remembered what Brant had given to me not only that year, but in all the years since we first met.

It started to turn around.

A lightning bolt of clarity struck me. If I dropped out, I would have no chance of winning. If I committed myself to finishing and gave it everything I had *every step that remained in the marathon,* there just might be a chance . . .

The battle was long, and the pain was intense. But, finally, with less than 2 miles to go, Thomas Hellriegel appeared in front of me. I caught him, passed him, and went on to my sixth—and final—Ironman Championship.

It was a great way to end my Ironman career. It also pointed out the importance of sitting down and examining your Energy Pie, evaluating where you are and what changes you might need to make. The answers might be different from what you expect.

A nine-day retreat with a shaman in Alaska is not standard triathlon training, but it was absolutely essential to my success. If Julie had not supported me with her commitment and given me the solitary time to train, I could not have prepared the way I did. There is no question in my mind that, without that support, I would not have won that race.

Julie and Mark: Freedom Julie: Freedom is finishing a mapped-out period at the end of a week or a race. It only lasts until the next mapped-out period begins. It's a breathing space between accomplishing one goal and setting the next.

Mark: Anytime your mind is quiet, anytime you accomplish a goal, anytime you see yourself clearly, anytime you share something with a friend or your family, anytime you take care of yourself—you are free. Anytime you forget about yourself in action, you give yourself freedom.

Part II

Get Going

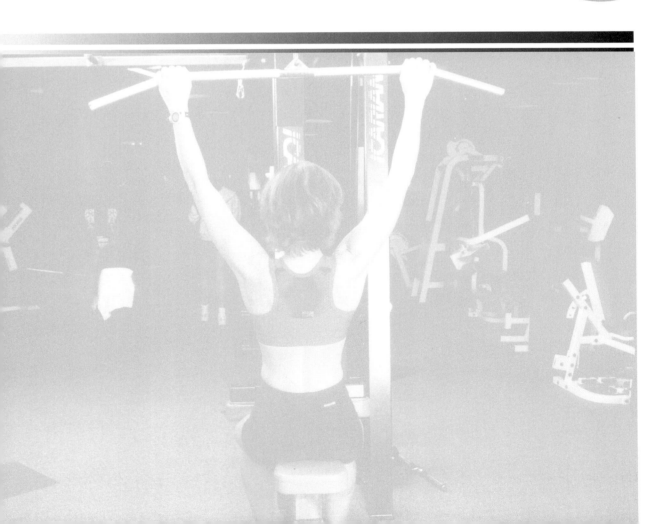

5 Time to Sweat

The goals have been set and you've committed the time and energy needed to work out. It's time to choose your athletic weapon, the fitness activities that will strengthen, sculpt, quicken, and transform your body and energy from where you are today up to new levels. The actual activity does not matter. Pick any form of movement where you can raise your heart rate and keep it elevated for twenty minutes or more. Walking, running, cycling, hiking, rowing, in-line skating, or pushing Junior in the Baby Jogger all count. What makes the difference is how fast, how long, and how often you exercise.

How Much Should I Work Out? The answer to this question depends on your goals and your current level of fitness. What is required in order to lose fifteen pounds over the next few months is very different from what it will take to win the Ironman Triathlon. Some studies indicate that as little as three twenty-minute workouts per week will cure what ails you. The reality is that there is probably no one alive who could achieve anything but the most benign goal on three twenty-minute workouts a week.

Julie: 45 Minutes a Day Forty-five minutes a day keeps me sane. It's my minimum to feel decent. It doesn't matter which exercises I choose. It can be a swim and a run or a long walk. If I got more, say around two to three hours a day, I would be ecstatic, but I rarely get that.

Part of the motivation for my exercise routine relates to eating. The more exercise I get, the more I can eat. I come from a family of great cooks, and we share a lot of incredible meals together. Exercising forty-five minutes a day, I have to be really conscious of eating smaller portions so I don't gain weight. Exercising two to three hours a day, I can relax about what I eat.

Rules of Thumb for Workout Lengths There is a limitless combination of workout lengths and frequencies, with no one right formula for everyone. Here are a few guidelines to help make the smart choice for you:

Longevity: If you are working out simply to live longer, expending about 2,000 calories per week through movement seems to provide the maximum benefit. This equates to about 3 miles a day of walking or running, or somewhere around three to four hours of working out every week.

Intellectual Balance: Work out as long as it takes for your mind to become quiet. The first part of any workout is usually spent thinking, solving problems, mulling over stresses, and so on. At some point, any resistance you may have had to working out or dilemmas that have been bugging you will cease to exist in your conscious mind. The next thing you are aware of is that you have not really been thinking about much at all. You have just been observing the world as you move your body. This state is meditation in motion and can be a very powerful way to regenerate and balance your body, mind, and spirit.

Practical: If you only have twenty minutes to work out, then the workout will be a twenty-minute workout. Don't stress out if you'd planned a forty- or fifty-minute workout. Just soak up all you can from those precious minutes you do have. Don't waste time getting your mind to quiet down or the workout will be done before you get to that regenerative state for your brain.

If you have only three workout slots per week, then that is the perfect amount for you at this time. If your life situation changes and more time opens up, then—if you choose—you can take advantage of the freedom.

Racing: Generally, when you are preparing for a race, one workout a week will be the designated endurance workout. This session should be about one and a half to three times the distance or time of your basic daily workout. If you can run about thirty minutes most days of the week, then your endurance workout should be somewhere between forty-five minutes and one and a half hours. Initially, choose the low end. Over time, you can increase the distance of the long workout to the upper end of the range. Ultimately, your long endurance workout should be between 75 percent to 150 percent of the distance or time you will be racing. If a 10K is your goal, your longest endurance workout leading up to it could be 5 to 10 miles. The choice of where to place yourself within these ranges will be up to you and your body's ability to absorb the workouts.

For racing, practical considerations of available time usually dictate the frequency of your workouts. Keep in mind that more is better up to the point where you begin to be irritable and

Cardiovascular Is King

There are two basic types of workouts. One is strength-based. The other is endurance- or cardiovascular-based. The main purpose of a strength workout is to build muscle mass and functional strength. The main benefit of doing an endurance or cardiovascular workout is to work your heart. If done correctly over time, these types of workouts together will change your body composition, increasing the flexibility of your muscles, joints, and even your rib cage—which will enable you to breathe easier. The cardiovascular workout will also help regulate the chemistry inside your body in a way that stabilizes blood sugar levels and promotes fat burning, which is a definite plus for most people.

Cardiovascular workouts require you to raise your heart rate, then hold it elevated during the bulk of the workout. Ironically, you probably won't have to go as hard as you thought you would to get the maximum results from your training.

burned out, or start to get minor injuries. These are all indications that you can no longer absorb the workouts you are doing and should back off some.

Physiological: Taking one or two days off will not affect the big picture of your fitness. In fact, often this is the break you need to absorb a hard block of training. But once you miss the third day in a row, your fitness will start to fall off. After a break of about two weeks, fitness starts to decline rapidly.

The good news is that the more consistent you are during the periods when you can be consistent, the quicker you will bounce back from any layoff. And remember, it's never too late to start!

Achieving Your Goal: If your current level of activity is not getting you the results you are after, you may need to increase the overall workout load to bring your workout schedule in line with what it will take to achieve your goal. If you want to run a marathon and your longest training workout is 5 miles, you may consider a modification of the program. If fifty pounds off is the goal, but only five have disappeared in the last three months, you may need to increase the frequency of those 3-mile walks you've been doing each week. Or keep the frequency the same but tag some extra distance onto the end of your normal route.

Mark, Julie, and Mats: Pleasure or Pain

Mark: Instead of thinking about pain, I usually look at any uncomfortable part of a workout as giving up my comfort. Once I surrender to that, there always comes some level of pleasure.

Julie: The most pleasurable part of a run is when it's over. The most painful part is waiting to get started. If there were a sensory word associated with procrastination, it would be *pain*.

Mats (on pleasure): Jokes and climbing the tree at home, that makes me happy. I feel happy to go for a hike to look for feathers.

Mark: Endurance

Endurance is, simply, the ability to continue. It is developed over time with repetition. It builds an innate knowl-

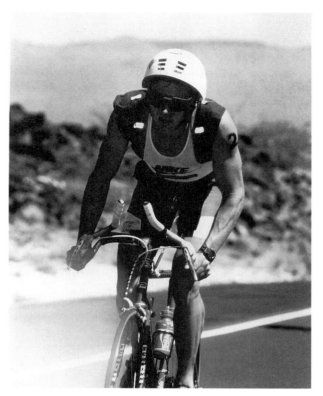

I should have known I was in trouble when my nose started bleeding during the 1987 Ironman bike ride. I just put it out of my mind and focused on the task at hand.

edge in your cells that may seem to slip away when you don't use it, but that comes back quickly when called upon.

Julie: Patience

Building endurance is a methodical, somewhat pain-free process. It just takes time and a lot of patience. Anyone can attain it. My philosophy is, if you can run a mile, you can run a marathon. The only difference between the first mile and the next twenty-five is having the patience to stick with an endurance program. And the best way to stick with it is to commit to a goal event somewhere in the future.

Anatomy of Your Anatomy in Motion

To understand how fast you need to work out, it helps to know what is going on inside that amazing machine called your body during motion. Your body uses two forms of stored energy to make muscles work: *fat* and

> ### AEROBIC WORKOUT:
> **Any workout where you are burning mostly fat as your source of energy.**
>
> ### ANAEROBIC WORKOUT:
> **Any workout where you are burning mostly carbohydrate as your source of energy.**

carbohydrate. In the reaction that breaks fat down into energy, more oxygen is used than in the reaction that breaks apart carbohydrate for energy. Understanding this simple difference in energy equations and learning to apply that knowledge will put you in the category of exercise guru. Here is an example of how this works.

Suppose your Great-Aunt Ophelia is going to be on *Jeopardy* later today. You are sitting around watching the tube in eager anticipation. Your energy needs for sitting still are minimal. And, since the energy requirements for lounging in the easy chair are low and the amount of oxygen you can take in is relatively high, your body will be burning mostly fat.

But you are bored because Auntie won't be on for half an hour and there is nothing that interests you on the television until then. So you decide to make a sandwich, which requires you to stand up and walk over to the refrigerator. Your energy requirement just went up. It took some energy to move those bones from the sofa to the kitchen, right? But unless you are extremely out of shape, you can still probably take in enough oxygen through your lungs and deliver it to the muscles via your bloodstream to use stored fat as your fuel for that small exertion.

Arriving at the Kenmore, you notice there is no mustard, and you just can't make your sandwich without it. It's time to get down to the convenience store several blocks away. You're not in a hurry. In fact, you are just killing time, so instead of driving, you decide to walk. Now even more energy is being used to move your body. Still, chances are that fat is the fuel of choice, since the energy requirement is not huge compared to your ability to take in oxygen.

You buy your Dijon and, on the way out of the store, you run into an old friend. You start talking, time passes, and, all of a sudden, you realize you will have to run to get back in time to see Aunt Ophelia on *Jeopardy.* Now you are testing the upper limits of your ability to take in enough oxygen quickly enough to break down fats to provide the energy needed for that run. Depending on your speed and level of fitness, you may even exceed it.

This brings you to option two for fuel. Without enough oxygen to burn fat, your body will switch over to carbohydrate burning. Remember that carbohydrates need less oxygen to be burned for energy than fats. Carbohydrates are like high-octane fuel for your body.

By sprinting, you make it back in time for the show. You think that, since you are back nestled into the Barcalounger with a low heart rate, you are back to burning fats. You are wrong. **Once you switch over to burning more carbohydrates than fat for energy, you do not go back to burning mostly fats for seven to nine hours, even though your heart rate is back down to what should be a fat-burning zone!**

Not only have you switched off your ability to burn fats for the next third of a day, but you have also done something else that is difficult for your body to undo. You have switched on your adrenal system. This is the place where your body stores up extra energy for times when it is needed. Do you remember the primitive fight-or-flight response? You turn on the adrenal system when you are afraid and need to flee danger. This system gets turned on during any type of stress, like being stuck in traffic and being twenty minutes late for an important meeting. Or worrying about a sick child—or parent. Any stress will do it, whether it's physical, mental, emotional, or environmental.

Do you feel better when you are relaxed or when you are stressed out? A different way to phrase the same question is, do you feel better when your adrenal system is being taxed and turned on or when it is regenerating and turned off? You may feel like a superhero when it is switched on, but there is a price for its use that can only be assessed once the adrenal system turns off. The price may be that you feel sleepy. You may also be irritable and unable to deal with anything else stressful—like noise (shut that kid up!). Over time, if you stress this system too frequently, you can become sick, injured, or have a heart attack and die.

Becoming a Fat-Burner

There are several reasons to develop your body's ability to burn stored fat. First, your reserves of fat are huge compared to the amount of stored carbohydrate in your body. In terms of endurance performance, burning as much fat as possible during a competition will spare precious glycogen (stored carbohydrate).

Why do you want to spare glycogen? Once you run out of it, your body stops working at a high level. In hard terms, you go from running to walking, and even that is painful. The only way to get going again is to ingest more carbohydrates. This may sound easy. Just slug down a Coke, right? Unfortunately, there may not be a convenience store nearby when you need one—and even if there is, it takes time for your body to assimilate the sugars and get them to your muscles. If your body can be more efficient, you'll go farther faster on less.

The improvement you can gain from increasing fat-burning efficiency is huge compared to the improvement in performance you will get from increasing carbohydrate-burning efficiency. Another way to look at it is that burning fat determines the size of your internal athletic engine. The more efficient you are at tapping into and utilizing the reserves of fat, the bigger your engine. Increasing your ability to burn carbohydrate only fine-tunes that engine.

Another reason being an efficient fat burner is a plus for health is that workouts in the fat-burning heart-rate ranges put less stress on your body and its adrenal system. It helps balance out the chemistry inside your body for optimal health.

No matter what your ultimate goal is, whether it's to lose sixty pounds or to win the Ironman, the application of this type of training is the same. Only the amount of time you spend training varies. And it enables you to get the most fitness out of the time you put in.

Johnny Workaholic and the Workout Neurotic

Johnny wanted it all: a great job, a loving family, and a toned body without the layer of fat most of his contemporaries have. His life was scheduled, booked, and overbooked, but somehow he seemed to make it all work. In fact, he was the envy of many a workout wannabe because he fit in his 5-mile run every day even if he had to sprint the entire way.

His coworkers just couldn't see how he kept his energy level so high. He didn't even drink coffee (no gigantic Starbucks cup in the morning for Johnny). And he seemed to survive on virtually no sleep.

Well, one day Johnny didn't come back from his 5-miler. The rumors started up immediately. He must be interviewing for a new position with a competitor. He's probably having an affair with his personal trainer. Several hours later, the office found out that he had had a heart attack during his run and was hauled off to the ER. The only interview he was having was with a cardiac specialist.

On the surface, Johnny appeared to be doing the right things. A closer look revealed that he was not really on the right track. Those crammed-in runs at maximum heart rate were shifting his metabolism into carbohydrate-burning mode every day, which in essence made it almost impossible for his body to develop the ability to burn fat. While Johnny didn't appear fat, there was a significant amount of it building up around his heart.

What about all those sleepless nights? They were a function of his overtaxed adrenal system, which basically never shut down. The combination of a stressful job and workouts that turned his adrenal system on meant he never gave himself a chance to regenerate. He didn't drink coffee because his adrenal system kept him as wired as if he'd had a gallon of it. He was out of balance.

Nature had to force Johnny to balance. Over time, he readjusted his schedule to be realistic, which reduced his work stress. He bought a heart-rate monitor to make sure he didn't overdo it when he worked out. The result was that he actually got the sleep he needed at night, his kids didn't get on his nerves, and that last ten pounds that he just couldn't lose before melted away because his body could finally burn fat.

Buy a Heart-Rate Monitor, Then Read On The only way to make sure you stay in your fat-burning range is to use a heart-rate monitor. It gives you instantaneous feedback about what is going on inside your body. Most people who don't work out with a heart-rate monitor work out too fast all the time. It's the "No pain, no gain" mentality. Even those who think they are being conservative and follow the rule of thumb that says you are aerobic as long as you can hold a conversation are often training at too high a heart rate to burn fat.

How fast a workout should be done is based upon your heart rate and your current level of fitness. In general, a fit person will be able to exercise at a higher heart rate before switching over to carbohydrate burning than an unfit person. So let us give you a formula that will determine the maximum heart rate you can exercise at before you make that switch from fat burning to mostly carbohydrate burning.

Mark: Heart Rates People who are very aerobically fit do not have very high maximum heart rates. Very unfit people, on the other hand, do have high heart rates. As a swimmer, my maximum heart rate was around 220. As a triathlete, it was about 178. The major difference was the change from training just the anaerobic system to training both the carbohydrate-burning and the fat-burning systems.

My dad's wife, Carole, is a classic example of the positive impact aerobic training can have. In her twenties and thirties, she never worked out and had a resting heart rate in the high 90s. She assumed that her heart rate was

Maximum Aerobic Heart Rate (MAHR)

Start with 180 and subtract your age. Take this number and correct using the following guidelines:

- Subtract another 10 beats for being a couch potato, or

- Subtract another 5 beats for being a recreational weekend athlete, or

- Leave the number alone for an athlete who has trained consistently three or more days per week for several years, or

- Add 5 beats for an athlete who has trained at a high level for several years.

- Now add 5 beats if you are either over sixty or under twenty.

The number you end up with will be your maximum aerobic heart rate (MAHR). If you exercise below this heart rate, you will burn fat for energy. If you exercise above this number, you will burn carbohydrate. Both systems are important, but the fat-burning system is the one that takes the longest and is the most difficult to develop.

genetically that fast, and there was nothing she could do to lower it.

Then she started running and lifting weights. Her resting heart rate is now in the 60s and 70s because her body can utilize fat as an energy source. She is more aerobically fit and significantly healthier. It's a total success story due to exercise.

Training Your Heart How can you get faster if you are training at a heart rate below your maximum? For illustration, let's say that it takes one fat-burning enzyme one second to break down one fat molecule to release enough energy to contract one muscle cell. In January, suppose you've only got one of these fat-burning enzymes in your body. This means that every second you will be able to contract one muscle cell.

Over the next several months, you train your body at aerobic heart rates, which in turn stimulates the production of fat-burning enzymes. By March, you will have more of these enzymes working together to convert fat into energy—say a thousand. This means that every second you can now convert a thousand fat molecules into energy that in turn contracts a thousand muscle cells. This translates into a faster athlete at the same heart rate.

You have just become an enzymatic wonder!

Mark: Aerobic and Anaerobic Workouts

I was a swimmer growing up. Every workout was a fast, anaerobic session. You could physically do this because there is not much tissue damage when you swim, which is very different from weight-bearing exercises like running. So when I entered triathlons in 1982, I tried to directly apply the way I trained as a swimmer to the sports of cycling and running.

Since I was trying to be a top-level competitor, I knew I was going to have to run around 5:15 minutes per mile in my short races, *after* swimming and cycling. I naturally thought that to do such a feat I needed to train at that pace—at least for a mile or two during every run workout. How could I do it in a race if I didn't do it all the time in my training?

Wrong! I had good results from all the fast training, but very slow recovery and lots of niggling injuries. Fortunately, in 1983 I was introduced to a man named Phil Maffetone, who was training some world-class athletes. All his training programs were based on basic heart rate rules. Phil told me initially to do the bulk of my workouts under 155 beats per minute, which he said would develop my aerobic system more fully. He said the speed work would come later.

Under some duress, I strapped on a primitive heart-rate monitor and took off for a run. I was shocked. I had to run about an 8:15 mile or slower pace to keep my heart rate from skyrocketing over the 155 barrier Phil had set. I had almost no ability to convert fat into energy.

So there I was, Mr. Ironman triathlete, training at a pace that was three minutes a mile slower than I was accustomed to and three minutes a mile slower than I knew I would need to go in a race to be competitive.

Swallowing my ego was the hardest part, but I kept at it. That 8:15 mile at 155 beats per minute slowly got faster. About a year and half later, I was back down to almost a 5:15 mile at a heart rate of 155 beats per minute! I was an aerobic machine.

From there, I combined both aerobic and anaerobic workouts to maximize the benefits from the heart-rate monitor. My racing improved, my consistency in workouts greatly improved, and my recovery happened virtually overnight from even the toughest workouts.

Julie: Heart-Rate Monitors

I have two theories about using a heart-rate monitor. If you run with a partner who is equal to or below your level and it's a conversational run, then you are probably running aerobically. If you are with someone faster, you need to wear the monitor or you will probably be running too hard. Heart-rate monitors are an objective voice that most likely will tell you to slow down, and occasionally to speed up.

Let's Get Going

Now, choose your exercise, strap on the heart-rate monitor, and go. If you are like most people, your first time out of the blocks with a heart-rate monitor on may be a shock. Keeping your heart rate below your Maximum Aerobic Heart Rate (MAHR) will probably make the workout seem too easy. This is only a function of your lack of aerobic fitness, which in many ways is a marker for your level of health.

Start out slowly, then over about ten to fifteen minutes, work your heart rate up to within 20 to 30 beats of your MAHR *without going over it*. Hold your heart rate in this range for the bulk of your workout, and voilà! You have worked your aerobic fat-burning system without stimulating your adrenal system or shutting off fat burning in favor of burning carbohydrate.

Improvements in fitness for a person who is totally out of shape happen by leaps and bounds. Improvements in fitness for the finely tuned athlete happen in almost imperceptible increments over painfully long periods of time.

MAPping Your Way Training by heart rates is not especially good for your ego in the short run. Slowing down is usually not equated with improvement. Even over time, it is difficult to "feel" your heart rate as a function of perceived effort. Dehydration, over- or undertraining, high ambient temperatures, or a low-grade illness all affect your heart rate, making it higher than your perception of effort would indicate.

You can monitor your progress by doing what Phil Maffetone calls a Maximum Aerobic Pace (MAP) Test. It is easiest to do this test at a running track in the following manner:

- Go to the track and warm up for 10–15 minutes, gradually increasing your effort until your heart rate is within 20–30 beats of your MAHR.

- Once you hit that heart rate, continue running and time a mile at your MAHR without going over it.

- The mile time will be your MAP.

- Repeat this test every two to three weeks. With consistent training in the aerobic zone, your pace will gradually get faster at the same heart rate.

Eventually, you will do the test and see that the pace is slower than the previous one. This is an indication that you have gotten all the benefit you are going to get for the time being by training aerobically. If you are interested in continuing to get faster, it is time to do some anaerobic work, which will require you to do one or two workouts per week where you elevate your heart rate above your MAHR.

- Continue to do the MAP test during this anaerobic speed phase. You should see your MAP time get faster until you reach another plateau and then a slowing of the test time. This indicates that it's time to go back to doing strictly aerobic heart-rate workouts.

Young people often get the maximum benefit from a block of aerobic training as indicated by their MAP track test in as little as four to six weeks. It may take as long as six months of consistent anaerobic work before they see a slowing of the MAP test that would indicate it is time to go back to aerobic training.

Older people can improve for up to six months before they see their MAP test slow down when doing a block of aerobic training. However, when they do anaerobic training, they may see the switch indicator during a MAP test after as little as four to six weeks.

Julie: Plateaus Plateaus are tough because even though you are working hard, there aren't any visible signs of improvement. And your first reaction is to work even harder, which may not be the answer to taking your fitness to the next level. It's somewhat like getting a promotion—you have to put in the time before the next one comes. If you are riding out a plateau, focus on the positive side, which is that you are at one of the points you've been shooting for. It can also be a time to experiment with different training techniques. Logically, if you've reached one plateau, you have all the tools to get to the next one. Just be patient and try to enjoy the view.

Mark: Balance During my career as a professional triathlete, I saw a lot of people who were extremely physically fit, but who were still not happy in their lives. Their spirit seemed weak or sick—out of balance. The time I spent studying Huichol shamanism with my teacher, Brant Secunda, was my way of paying attention to my emotional and spiritual health, then integrating those with my physical health. It brought me into a more finely tuned balance that enabled me to go out and tackle the challenges that most tested me, like the Ironman. My results are living proof of what can happen when this type of integration begins to happen.

Several years ago, I was able to give back to

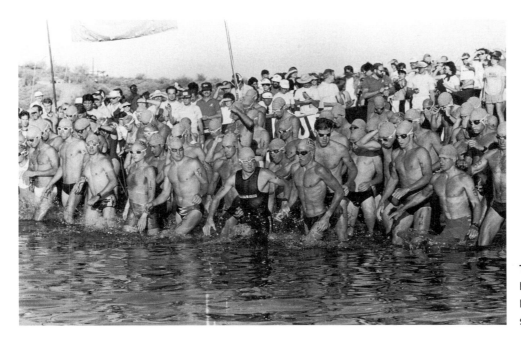

The multisport lifestyle builds balanced bodies better than any single sport can.

Brant in a small way for all his teaching and help. After his twelve-year apprenticeship in Mexico to become a shaman, he was in great physical shape. But slowly, in the years that followed, he gained fifty pounds. So in December of 1997, I helped Brant start a balanced training program that combined aerobic work with time in the gym doing strength training. It was designed to fit the needs of today's demanding work environment and his heavy lecturing and seminar schedule. We also restructured his diet, moderately decreasing the amount of carbohydrates and increasing the amount of protein.

Brant started by walking and jogging six days per week. Initially, he did this without a heart-rate monitor, letting his body set the pace. The transformation was amazing. By spring a year later, he had lost about thirty pounds of fat and gained a significant amount of lean muscle. Then he hit a plateau.

At that point, we figured out his MAHR, he strapped on the heart-rate monitor, and he went for an aerobic run. He had to slow things down slightly from the pace he had been running. He asked, "Am I going fast enough? It seems so slow!"

When he ran without the monitor, after twenty minutes it got very difficult to maintain his pace. With the heart-rate monitor on, keeping his heart rate below his MAHR, he was able to go over forty minutes and he felt refreshed from his workouts instead of tired. A short time after that, his weight was down to ideal, nearly fifty pounds below his starting weight just months before!

You Can't Have It Both Ways Why divide workouts up into two distinct categories—aerobic and anaerobic? Simply put, it is more difficult for your body to develop the fat-burning system than the glucose-burning anaerobic system. It is a harder system to stimulate. For example, let's say you go for a two-hour bike ride, spending the first 1:45 in your aerobic fat-burning range. Then one of your buddies gets the group going and you go into your anaerobic heart range for five minutes near the end of the ride.

What happens? You have just turned off your fat-burning system, and your body can't go back to full fat-burning mode for seven to nine hours. Also, your body has been given the choice of developing either fat- or carbohydrate-burning capability. It will choose the carbohydrate mode every time. So even though you spent the vast majority of the workout in the aerobic range, your body will view it as an anaerobic session and will only develop that system. You will also require the additional recovery time that goes with an anaerobic workout.

For recovery, aerobic is king. An anaerobic workout, one where you take your heart rate up above the MAHR into the carbohydrate-burning zone, tends to leave you feeling trashed, like you really did something. Slowing the workout down even a few beats to stay within the aerobic range often leaves you feeling fresher than when you started out.

Mark: It's There for You Some people think this kind of training is ridiculous. A lot of athletes say they do not need a heart-rate monitor to tell what their heart rate is. I spent fourteen years using a heart-rate monitor, playing with it every single workout and doing every kind of mind game to see if I could guess, and I know you can't be accurate all the time.

I personally thought it would be boring to train with a heart-rate monitor. I thought I would be a slave to it. I wanted a bust-loose kind of feeling. But I found over time that it was one of my most enjoyable training partners. I made it a game to see if I had to go slower when I went up a hill. Most of the time, I was thankful it was telling me it was time to slow down a bit.

Another plus to a heart-rate monitor is that it does not talk back to you. It does not tell you stupid jokes. It does not ask you personal questions you don't want to answer. Like a good dog, it's there for you.

> *Studies have shown that people who begin an exercise program with high-intensity workouts are far more likely to quit than those who adopt a moderate approach.*

Getting to Know Your Body Your body changes with the speed of a blooming tree. Day to day, you may not see the difference, but as weeks go by, there's a major transformation. It takes trust. Getting to the point where fitness does not leave you sore is an organic process your body goes through. Changes are subtle and take place over time. If you can be motivated to stay relatively consistent over a long enough period of time, you will make those breakthroughs. Once you make those breakthroughs, you will be amazed. You will gain fitness and confidence that will never go away.

Mark: Feeling the Difference When I started training each year, my pace at 150 bpm (heartbeats per minute) would be about seven minutes per mile. That pace changed and got faster at about one half to three fourths of a second per mile per day. Put in different terms, this meant that on Monday I would run a mile at 150 BPM in seven minutes. On Tuesday, at the same heart rate, I could run the mile in about 6:59.5 minutes.

There is no way I could perceive that small a difference. By the end of the week, if I was lucky, I would be clipping along at about a 6:55 per mile. It is still extremely doubtful that I could distinguish this small a change. In fact, that quicker mile probably felt slower because I was in better shape.

Later in the season, I would run the mile at 150 bpm around a 5:20 to 5:25 pace. Now, that difference I could *feel.* Over time, if you keep at it, you will notice the difference.

From Flab to Fit If you do virtually nothing now, your initial improvement from working out will be dramatic. The workouts will be new, the change in your body will happen quickly, and you will feel as if nothing can stand in the way of your goal of personal body transformation. It can be intoxicating.

At first, you may feel a little like a foreigner in your own skin. Your body is simply going through changes. Don't worry about being a little sore. If you think about it, it is not really all that painful. Often the sensations of pumping life through a changing body get confused with pain. This is just a byproduct of moving new parts of your body.

As long as the pain cannot be pinpointed in one place, keep going. If the pain can be pinpointed, like in a knee or ankle, then it's time to pack it in for the day because you may be flirting with injury.

You will never see that great a gain again. You go through different levels. The initial excitement you get motivates you and galvanizes your commitment. But then you hit a plateau, and suddenly another trip to the gym doesn't sound so much like your cup of tea. This is normal.

The body does not change on a linear scale. If you start to lose momentum, don't lose faith. A lot of people give up on the program during plateaus. Say you are working out for weight loss and you lose fifteen pounds pretty quickly, then get stuck. With performance goals, plateaus happen all the time. You steadily improve your times at the track, and then you can't get any faster for a month or two.

Plateaus are interesting. They can mean your body is building up a critical mass of fitness and all you need to do is keep on the current program. Or a plateau can mean you need to correct something. Assess your fitness with a MAP test. It might be time to switch the phase you are in.

Analyze your diet and see if it is in line with your current level of commitment to your workouts. A junky diet does not support a great workout program. If all else fails, look at your life. If all you can see is stress, stress, and more stress, change the things within your control that you can to reduce your stress level.

How to Do the Workouts All workouts should start out slowly. Leave your stretching for after. Unless you are extremely stiff, it is much better to warm up slowly, letting the stiffness of your body determine the pace. Then, as the blood starts moving and the internal systems start working, your pace will pick up naturally. You can avoid a lot of injuries simply by starting out very, very slowly.

After the warm-up period, you can continue to work your heart rate up to get within the training range. For aerobic workouts, improvements will be quickest when more time is spent training near your MAHR without going over. It's your choice, depending on the energy level you have on any given day and how much of that workout you are willing to push to stay in the upper level of the zone. However, as you get more aerobically fit, it will become increasingly difficult to keep your heart rate in the upper ranges for long periods of time, simply because you will be going so fast.

As a rule, in the beginning of a workout it will be difficult to get your heart rate up. As the workout goes on, especially for longer ones, you may actually need to slow your pace down to keep your heart rate below the aerobic maximum. This is normal. If the workout is to be aerobic, do whatever it takes to keep your heart rate below your aerobic maximum.

For anaerobic workouts, the objective is to get your heart rate above the aerobic maximum. During a speed session, it may be difficult to get above your MAHR for the first few intervals. Then, just like in the aerobic workouts, it will become easier to elevate the heart rate as you go. Here, however, you don't need to worry about your heart rate getting high—that is the objective. You are trying to tax the anaerobic system to increase muscle recruitment, stimulate carbohydrate burning, and develop neurological firing.

A third type of workout is designed for recovery. These are the be-good-to-yourself workouts. They are just as important as any hard session you do. During recovery workouts, it's important to keep your heart rate at least 20 beats below your MAHR. This helps your body flush byproducts out of the tissues and put energy back into your body instead of taking it out. Even though you are going slowly, you should still be thinking about your form, which will continue to pattern your muscle firing in a very efficient way.

Every workout should be approached with the goal of building your speed throughout the workout, especially during interval workouts. Your first interval should be the slowest, the last the fastest.

Mark: Peace A little fatigue is normal; a lot is not. It's important not to confuse being relaxed with being fatigued. We are a caffeinated, revved-up society. Expending physical energy is a way to regain a balance of energy output that matches our normal need to expend energy. When we do that, we are at peace—which a lot of people might see as fatigue.

Julie: Fatigue I actually love the feeling of fatigue. I love dropping into bed at night tired from a good workout. For example, when lifting weights, the goal is to reach muscle fatigue. This means you build new muscle tissue and recruit more muscles to do the work. You can't go to the next level until you can fatigue yourself on a short-term basis. To reach a very high level of fitness, there are going to be periods of fatigue, which will make you stronger when you recover from them.

Which Exercise Is for Me? No one exercise works for everyone. Running is the savior for one person and a nightmare for someone else. If you don't like the activity you are currently doing, try something else. There is one out there that will agree with both you and your body.

Julie: Simplicity What I like best about running is that it's simple. You can do it anywhere. It's a real no-brainer. Also, it's the one that gets me sweating the fastest, and sweating always makes me feel better.

Walking When you walk, you use very fine muscles that normally don't come into play when you run. Walking also develops your body's ability to flush tissues of metabolic byproducts. When you do go faster, like during a run, your recovery period between each step is quicker.

Francesco Moser attributed his world record for cycling to walking. He walked for forty-five minutes to an hour after he ate dinner every day. The walking helped to digest food and take

> *Try in-line skating with an old pair of ski poles. It gets your upper body involved, too.*

it out of the stomach into muscle so it didn't turn to fat. He also developed that ability to flush the muscle.

You end up being a faster runner or cyclist when you develop the body's ability to flush muscles out and remove waste. It also improves general life health. Walking is one of the best exercises you can do. Walk with a little more purpose than a stroll, however. Put some intent into it, just shy of breaking into a slow jog, and then you really get the benefits.

Mark: Fast Walking Earlier this year, I took my car in to get it detailed. The place I had to take it was about 5 miles from my house. I thought it would take twenty minutes, like the cheap car wash I normally go to. The guy said, "Come back in about five hours." I looked at him. I was 5 miles from home, Julie was gone, and I was going to have to either hang out at the auto detailers or do the unthinkable and walk home.

I decided to walk. Fast walking. The next day, my entire body felt strong from that unplanned adventure.

Tennis It would be a stretch to consider tennis an aerobic exercise. Most motion happens in quick spurts and it is difficult to keep your heart rate elevated for any period of time. And most of those movements are bursts that probably qualify as anaerobic movement.

Basketball This could be aerobic, but you might be going too fast and hard to keep it below the aerobic threshold. I don't think Michael Jordan has any excess body fat, but then he works out for hours every day. A weekend game of B-ball doesn't really cut it as an aerobic staple.

Mountain Biking This can be aerobic, depending on your effort. On steep trails, it can be difficult to regulate your heart rate. It can become a full anaerobic effort just to keep from falling over. If you are in the anaerobic phase of your training, go for it. But to build the size of your engine, stick to the gentle rollers.

Swimming This one is difficult to regulate because most monitors don't work too well in the pool. One way around this is to plop yourself into an easy lane while getting in shape and swim with moderate efforts, checking your pulse at the end of each swim. Then as you get in better shape, move over into the stud lanes with the sharks who like to swim fast all the time.

Versaclimbers, Stairmasters, and Treadmills Lots of people like the gym because they don't have to deal with traffic, darkness, or hot and cold weather. With equipment that works your cardiovascular system like treadmills and rowing machines, plus strength equipment, a health club is like a fitness Disneyland.

One of the latest innovations is indoor cycling, something like aerobics on a bike. Someone leads the class to music and the workout is done on a modified stationary bicycle. It can be a very intense workout. The only difficulty is keeping your heart rate within the range that is right for you. However, factors of group moti-vation and your happiness quotient from the workout sometimes override the scheduled program.

Base Sports You may do any number of activities—basketball, skiing, rock climbing—but you're unlikely to be able to do them frequently enough to get in shape. Using a base of exercises like running, swimming, and cycling plus strength work can make those golden moments on the slopes or on the court just that much better.

Tips

- Never leave the house without a note stating when you left and when you will be back.

- Never run in the dark without a partner.

- Always wear a hat to protect you from the sun.

- Make sure you are not low on calories before you start your workout.

- Hydrate, hydrate, hydrate—drink sixteen to thirty-two ounces of water per hour of exercise, especially in the heat.

6 Pump It Up— Weight Training

Strength training is about changing your body composition. Strength adds to everything you do athletically. It will keep you from losing muscle mass, it fights gravity as far as reshaping your body, and it complements your daily life. It's the very best thing you can do—especially for anyone over thirty. In fact, you can retain almost 90 percent of your strength up until about age sixty if you put your muscles to work.

Strength training is the most commonly overlooked tool available for improving overall health. Yes, weight training builds muscle. It can also lower cholesterol, reduce blood pressure, improve glucose metabolism, and burn body fat. Weight training can muscle up your heart, thickening the walls and making it a more efficient pump.

The good news is that most of the benefits from a weight program can be yours for the low price of two extra hours of working out per week. In fact, with a well-executed strength program, you can effectively cut 10 percent to 25 percent off your aerobic exercise regime and come up with the same or better results!

Mark: Intimidation For my first nine years racing as a triathlete, I didn't lift one weight—and there was one very real but ridiculous reason I didn't. Gyms intimidated me. I lacked any knowledge about how to lift weights and a secure enough body image to set foot inside a gym. I knew I wouldn't impress anyone by bench pressing an empty bar.

So there I was, Mr. Ironman Champion, totally intimidated to go into the weight room. The people in the health club, well, their bodies looked different from mine. I did not fit in with the average physique in the gym. When you don't blend in, you stand out. Sometimes standing out is what you are after, but I like to blend in.

It was pretty silly, really. Nobody cared what I did or did not look like. If someone did notice me, it was a momentary glance and a quick, "Oh, he is skinny." I let my negative "gym image" hold me back from doing something I should have done years before.

But by the time I was thirty-three, my results were beginning to suffer, and I knew the only reason was because I wasn't as strong as I had been. So I swallowed my ego and started working with one of the best personal trainers

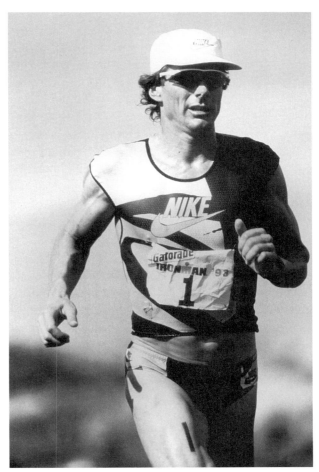

The hard part about being the defending champion? You are the target and everyone is gunning for you.

in the world, a woman named Diane Buchta.

She was there for every single weight workout I did over the course of a year. She took me through a whole cycle, adapting my body to weights. I was very sore the first few times, but ultimately it paid off. I had perhaps my best year racing ever. At the end, I was still not pushing around enough metal to raise eyebrows. But I didn't care. I had faced my fear.

> *It can take a year to put on seven to ten pounds of lean muscle mass.*

Julie: Benefits of Lifting I work out in the gym about two hours every week to maintain my strength. There are some really nice benefits from lifting. Any good weight program is going to reshape your body like no other form of working out. The results can be dramatic in eight to ten weeks of weight training.

Keep in mind that there is a fundamental difference between weight loss and body composition change. Don't fall into the "black hole" of jumping on a scale every day. Weight training made me focus on body composition instead of weight loss. Making it a goal to reshape through gaining muscle mass is very different from doing it through weight loss. The first time I tried it, I ended up losing eight to ten pounds in as many weeks!

Now that I am forty and have a child, I need to maximize my workout time. I have been able to maintain the strength I had ten years ago from hours of swimming, cycling, and running in two weight workouts per week.

Enjoy the Hidden Benefits Who needs strength? Everyone. Just think about a day in your life: You get out of bed first thing in the morning. That is a sit-up plus half a squat, a move that is repeated anytime you stand up from a sitting position: out of a chair, the car, off the sofa to get another cold one. Now consider a load of groceries. They don't just walk into the house on their own. Someone has to lift them and, depending on how you do it, this requires strength in your back, biceps, and shoulders, plus all the leg muscles necessary to walk the distance from the garage to the kitchen.

Anyone have kids? Caring for Junior turns into a full-body weight workout—lifting, lowering, carrying, and holding. As they grow older, children are defined by their toys, ranging from a mere ball up to a thirty-pound bike, in-line skates, and more groceries. Dirty clothes? How do they get from the hamper to the laundry room? In an ideal world, they arrive in the arms of the heir, but probably you are the one who does the honors in a rush to get the load in before some other task needs to be done that requires your hidden strength.

Practicalities aside, there are natural reasons to take up strength training as well. It's a matter of "use it or lose it." A strength program helps prevent injury because your joints and tendons stay strong beyond what we consider normal, and you have less chance of ending up with an accidental twist or strain from normal life.

The older you get, the more important flexibility becomes. New activities make you stiff and sore. That soreness is only partially from a lack of flexibility, however. Behind it all is a basic lack of strength that used to just be there.

Mark: Spiritual Strength Physical strength is inextricably tied up with mental and spiritual strength. To me, the important strengths are resilience from all that life has to offer, persistence even when the goal may not seem attainable, and a willingness to surrender to whatever a situation or goal may require.

Physical strength is simply the ability to function the way we were meant to. With that power, there is self-confidence, the ability to move in the world without being overwhelmed by it, and the capacity to remain centered.

Julie: Making A Choice Strength is a lifelong pursuit. I used to take it for granted, but now I realize I need to nurture it. Strength needs to be a deliberate choice if it's going to be maintained. Aerobic exercise, good nutrition, and recovery support a solid strength program.

Strength workouts are one of the main forms of training Mark and I can do together.

The weights are different, but the exercises are exactly the same.

We can go together, lift at the same time and spot each other if necessary on heavier equipment. We can also do our sets of abdominals together (even though I outdo him by far in this part of the workout). Of all the sports we do, it's one of the easiest, least stressful ways to work out together.

After the age of thirty, men lose about 1 percent of their muscle mass each year.

Keeping Up Rocky Marciano, unbeaten heavyweight champion, found out the hard way. He got a serious back injury from lifting his child. Even the mighty can be laid low if they don't stay current with fitness and weight training.

When John Glenn, at the age of seventy-seven, made his historic return to outer space, one of the primary topics of research was the effect of weightlessness on his body. In a low-gravity environment, muscles atrophy at an alarmingly fast rate, along with other physiological changes associated with aging. In essence, a human in space is transformed into the equivalent of an inactive elder in the span of a few days.

Strength training triggers the release of human growth hormone (HGH), which in turn stimulates the development of lean muscle mass. Lean muscle is denser and requires more calories to maintain than fat. In other words, a person who weighs 160 pounds and whose body is composed of 40 percent fat will require fewer calories every day to maintain his or her weight than someone who is 160 pounds with a body fat percentage of only 10 percent.

Mark: Getting Stronger I had one goal from strength training, and that was to get my body stronger. I had no desire to gain maximum strength or become a mass of muscles. I was in the gym to develop enough strength to be able to do my other activities at their fullest capacity. I did this with about two hours a week of weight work.

During my first full year of strength training, I won the Triple Crown of multisport racing: Nice, Zofingen, and the Hawaii Ironman. I didn't just win them, either. I triumphed. I felt as if I had core strength to draw upon that was beyond anything I had experienced before.

Study This A long-term study was done on a group of runners who competed in the Boston Marathon. One group consisted of men and women who just ran for their exercise. The second group ran and did strength training. Both groups were measured for lean muscle changes over a twenty-year period. The group who just ran lost measurable amounts of lean muscle mass. The ones who supplemented their running with strength work maintained their lean muscle mass over the same period.

Most of what we consider to be normal aging is really only a lack of exercise, flexibility work, and strength. Falling down, brittle bones, dropping hormone levels, joint pain—all of these are due to inactivity more than the aging process. Every basic movement you do in life will be easier and enhanced if you are little bit stronger.

Research has shown that most of the benefits from strength training are realized by doing two overall body workouts per week, with each workout exercise done in two sets of 12 to 15 repetitions. More than two days a week or more than fifteen repetitions on each set give only slightly greater improvements in strength. Depending on the rest of your workout load, doing more than two strength days per week may actually *decrease* your overall strength because of an inability to recover fully between sessions.

Julie: Using a Coach When I first started lifting weights, I wasn't intimidated by the thought of being a woman in what can be a very testosterone-soaked environment. My initial fears were about being out of shape, being in a foreign environment, and lacking any knowledge about how to use the equipment.

I hid behind loose clothes to overcome self-consciousness about my body. And I used a strength coach to help me learn how to use the equipment correctly. It took a few sessions, but eventually I felt comfortable with the machines and the workout. A strength coach can offer objective ideas about the places on your body that need extra attention, and offer solutions on how to transform them. The gym mirrors are brutal, but my strength coach pointed out how they let you see the muscles you are trying to isolate and help you exercise them properly. In my opinion, money spent on a strength trainer yields the biggest return on the time you invest at the gym.

Mark: We All Need It When you're done strength training, your body feels like you've tightened up the loose nuts and bolts. Over time, things shake loose. Aerobic training (running, walking, swimming) will do some to help your machine run more smoothly. But sooner or later you will need strength training. It's like giving a car a tune-up. You tighten all the bolts and make the suspension work just right.

The Strength Program During this entire program, there are a few critical keys to keep in mind.

• Taking a day off between sessions is essential. Lifting stimulates the muscles to grow. But the muscles actually grow when they're resting.

• Each exercise should be done to a count of two when the weight is lifted and a count of four when it is lowered. The only exception is during the final part of the program, the *chisel* phase. During this, lift *and* lower the weight to a count of two.

• Form is of utmost importance. Isolation of each muscle group is the goal.

• Breathe out as you lift a weight, in as you lower it. Holding your breath during a lift can send your blood pressure skyrocketing.

• Recent research indicates that a shorter rest between lifts—thirty seconds versus two to three minutes—seems to promote greater muscle growth.

• Warming up is extremely important in weight lifting. Try five to ten minutes of light exercise.

The strength program is divided up into four phases: *Adaptation, Endurance, Power,* and, finally, *Chisel.*

The Adaptation Phase *Adaptation* is the initial phase everyone goes through who has been away from the gym more than about two weeks. The goal is to adapt your body to the stress and motion of weight lifting. During this phase, each exercise is done for one set of 12 to 15 reps. Choose a weight so that you feel as if you could have done several more reps with good form at the end of each set. It will be time to go on to the next phase when you can do the routine without soreness. Generally this takes two to four weeks. By the end of this phase, you will start to feel the need to increase the weight so that you feel like you only had two or three repetitions left in you at the end of the set.

The exercises should be done in the following order for all phases:

1. LATERAL PULL-DOWNS

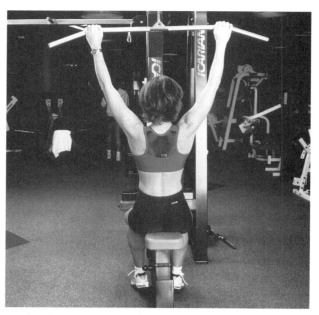

Beginning Position: Adjust knee brace so that legs are held in place by the padded bar when seated. Grasp bar with arms slightly wider than shoulder width. Keep thumbs on same side of bar as your fingers. The bar should be just slightly in front of your head. Push chest forward, arch lower back.

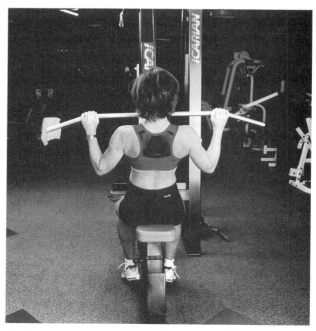

Ending Position: Upper body is rocked back slightly. Bar is in front of head at mid-shoulder level. Keep lower back arched, which will engage lats instead of chest.

2. LEG EXTENSION

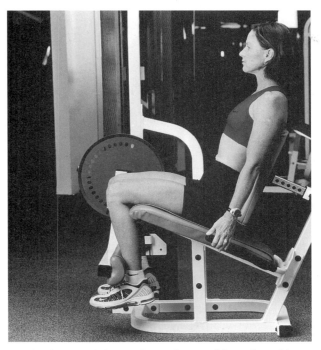

Beginning Position: Adjust shin pad length to hit comfortably above your ankle. Adjust backrest so knee pivots directly in line with same pivot point on the machine. Start point is with weights lifted just slightly off the stack.

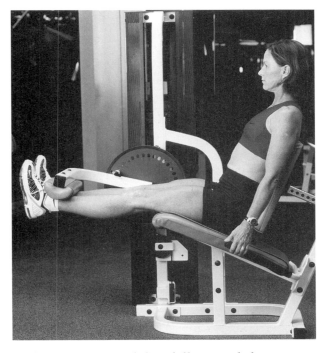

Ending Position: Both legs fully extended in straight line position.

3. LEG CURLS

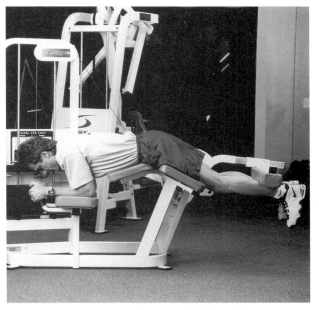

Beginning Position: Adjust padded leg lift to a position just above the ankle. Start with legs slightly bent (not straight).

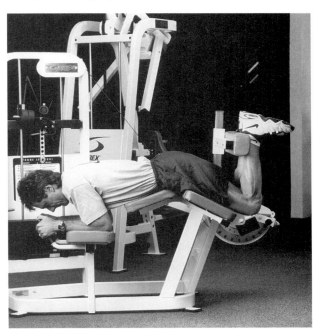

Ending Position: As fully contracted as possible without straining hamstrings. During lift, keep stomach on the pad at all times. Raising the stomach off the brace will engage the lower back instead of hamstrings.

4. BENCH PRESS

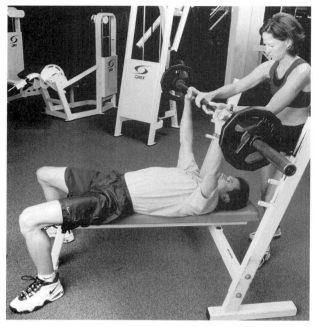

Beginning Position: Place hands just wider than shoulder width. Lift bar off support and position it above midchest. Spotter can have hands near bar for support if necessary. Spotter should have one hand below and one above bar.

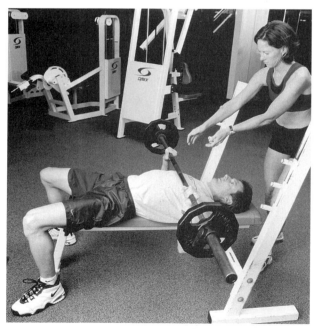

Ending Position: Stop the movement about an inch above midchest. Keep lower back on the bench at all times, especially during raise of the bar back up to the start position.

5. SQUATS

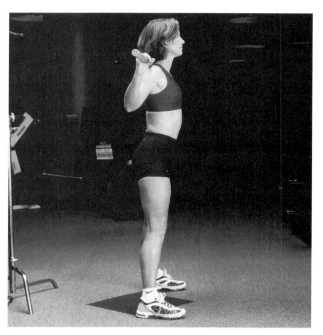

Beginning Position: Legs split slightly wider than shoulders. Arch lower back. Rest bar on upper back, not shoulders and neck. *Keep your body's weight over your heels during the entire exercise, not over your toes.*

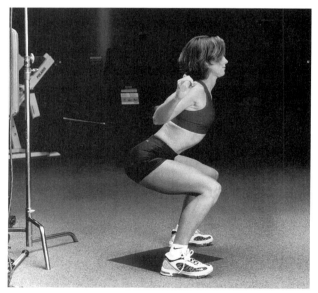

Ending Position: Butt is rocked back. Upper leg is parallel to floor. Knees should never extend out in front of toes. Extending your knees in front of your toes exerts a huge amount of pressure on them and can cause injury. If you have any knee pain, do not do this exercise. An alternate exercise is the leg press.

OR LEG PRESS

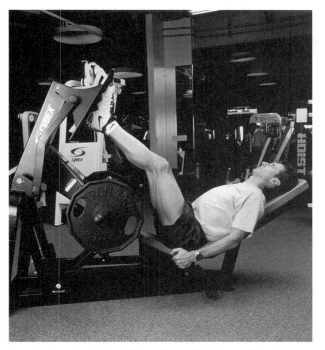

Beginning Position: Place feet slightly wider than shoulder width, with toes near upper part of foot plate. Keep knees from locking, just slightly bent.

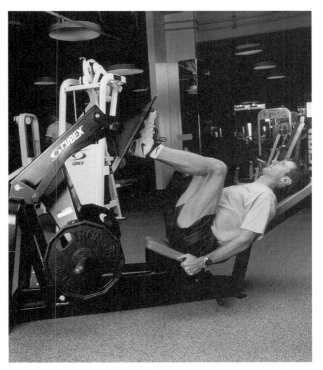

Ending Position: Lowered to a squat position, about the point where your knees would touch your chest. Keep lower back against seat.

6. DUMBBELL PULLOVER

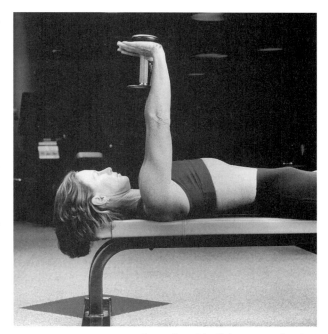

Beginning Position: Clasp dumbbell between both hands with arms straight.

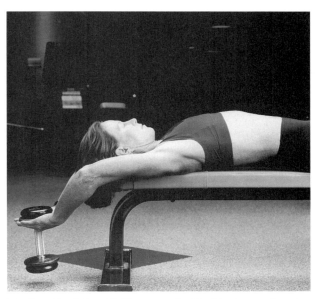

Ending Position: Fully extended behind your head, with weight touching floor if you are that flexible.

Special Note: Unlike all other exercises, during which you inhale on lowering the weight and exhale on the lift, in the Dumbbell Pullover you breathe out as you lower the weight behind your head, then inhale on the lift. This allows your rib cage to extend fully on the lowering phase.

7. BENT OVER ROW

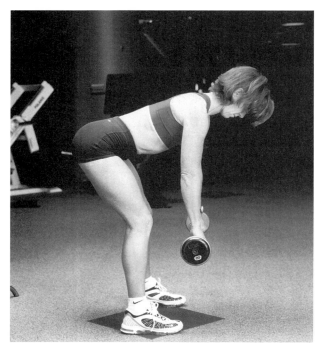

Beginning Position: Bend your knees, keep upper back straight and lower back slightly arched, and grasp bar with hands shoulder-width apart.

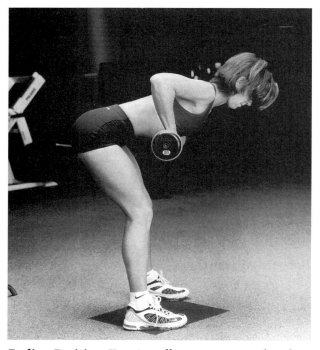

Ending Position: Keeping elbows up, stop when bar touches chest at midchest.

8. WALKING LUNGES

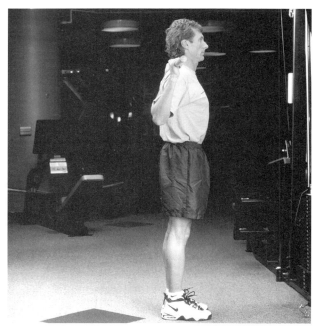

Beginning Position: Legs together, rest the bar comfortably on upper back.

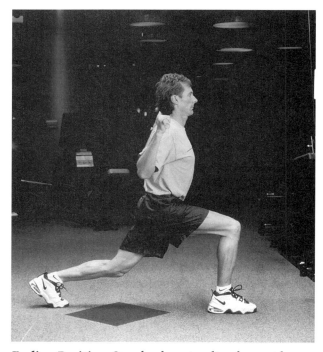

Ending Position: Step back, extending leg out behind. Returning to the starting position, drag the toes of the extended foot on the floor on the way back up to the neutral position.

9. SIDE LATERAL RAISES

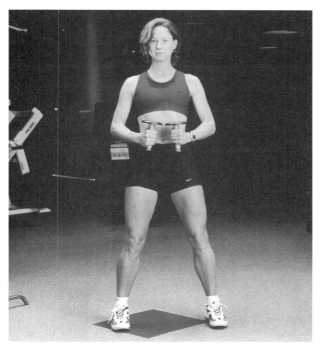

Beginning Position: Hold a weight in each hand, elbows even with the plane of your body and slightly extended away from your torso.

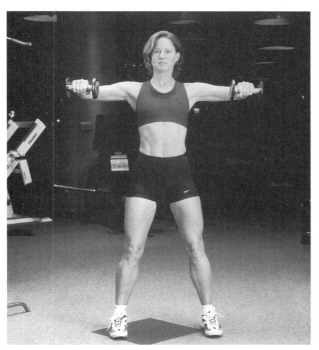

Ending Position: Extend arms out sideways, keeping elbows still in the plane of your body. Stop when upper arms are parallel to ground. Stop short of this position if you have any shoulder pain.

10. BICEPS

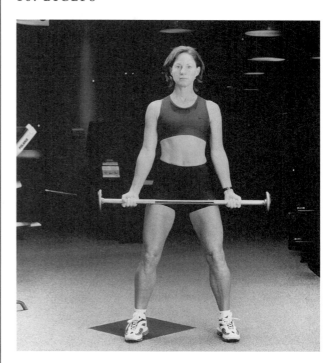

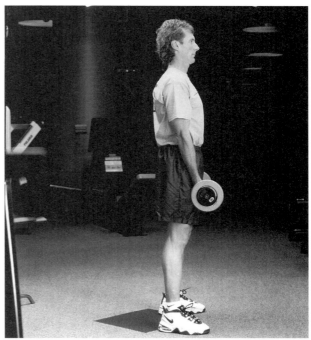

Beginning Position: Start with weight lowered, elbows tight against the side of your body and arms slightly bent (not with elbows locked).

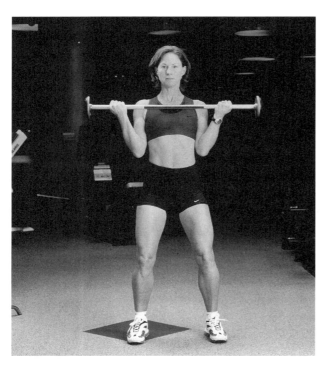

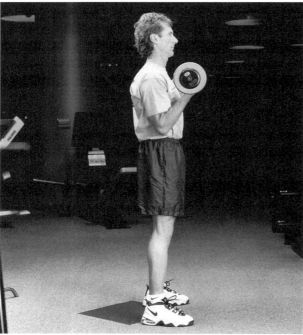

Ending Position: Arms contracted up, still supporting weight with your biceps (not resting in a locked position). Make sure to keep elbows locked tight against your side. Don't let them drift behind the plane of your body on the lift.

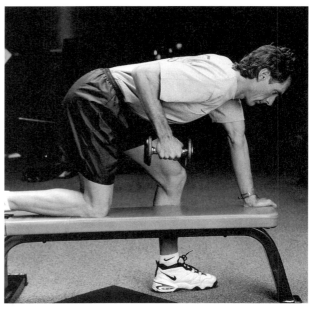

Beginning Position: Place one leg on the bench, the other foot on the floor. Support your upper body with the arm on the same side as the foot that is on the floor. Place the weight in the hand on the same side as the leg that is on the bench. Keep elbow tight against your side.

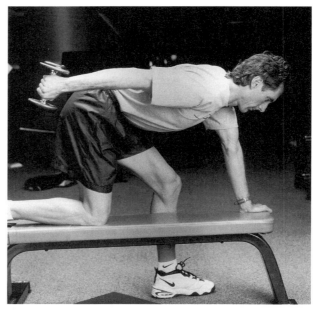

Ending Position: Extended back fully in straight position.

12. CALF RAISES

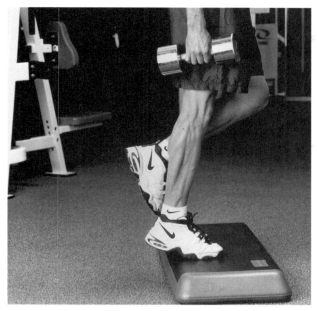

Beginning Position: Place one foot on a step and the other raised off the step just slightly. Hold the weight in the arm on the same side as the calf you are working.

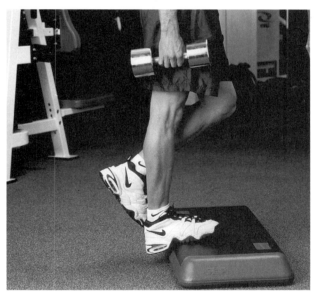

Ending Position: Lower heel until there is a moderate stretch on the calf muscle. Do not lower to a severe stretch point. This can cause the calf to cramp or rip.

Sit-ups

A note on all of the following sit-ups: Work all areas of the abdomen (lower, middle, and upper), but don't go crazy with abdominal exercises. It is important to strengthen this area because it helps with lower back problems, and it is the platform off which your body pushes during running. However, if you overdevelop your abdominals, you cannot breathe properly. Effective breathing comes from expanding your abdomen, not from raising your shoulders. If your abdominals are too developed, you cannot get a relaxed, deep breath. Our rule of thumb is no more than five minutes of moderate abdominal work per session.

13. LOWER ABDOMINAL SIT-UPS

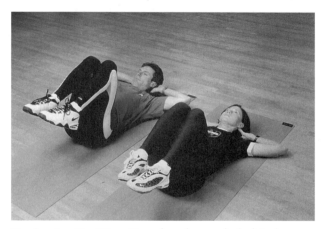

Beginning Position: Rest hands gently behind your head. Raise head off mat several inches without using hands to do it. Bring knees up to a neutral position above hips and let lower legs fall freely.

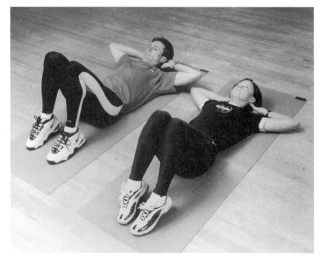

Ending Position: Tap feet on the floor. Keep lower back touching floor during entire lowering and raising of feet.

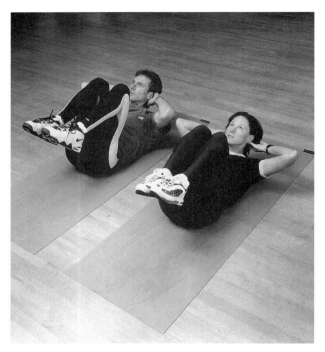

Beginning Position: Same start position as lower abs, except that upper body is raised up several inches off of the floor.

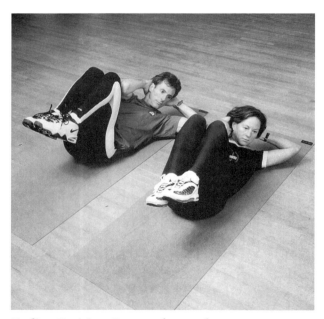

Ending Position: Same as lower abs.

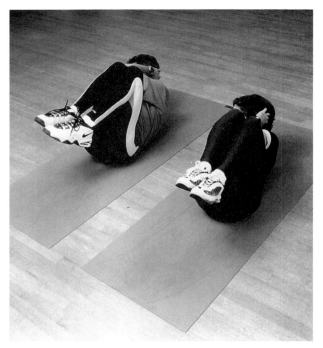

Beginning Position: Lower and midback are kept on the mat at all times. Upper back and knees are lifted, bringing your forehead close to your knees.

Ending Position: Knees are kept in same position, but upper back is lowered in a small motion. This is the famous crunch. The motion is short. You can lower the legs just several inches to accentuate the upper abs.

The Endurance Phase The next phase is *Endurance.* This phase lasts longer than Adaptation. Depending on your goals, you can do this phase year-round. If you have specific strength or racing goals in mind, the Endurance phase should be done for five weeks to three months before shifting into Power.

During the Endurance phase, you will do two sets of 12 to 15 reps. Choose a weight that allows you to complete the two sets knowing you could have done two to three more reps before failure. As your strength begins to go up, you will need to add weight to get the desired fatigue at the end of the second set.

Consider the effort to be an "aerobic" one, even though there is no such thing as an aerobic weight workout. However, try not to use so much weight that each exercise becomes a major burn session. That will come in the next phase.

The Power Phase Next up is *Power*. This phase is where the largest improvements in strength are made. However, you might experience some sluggishness in your aerobic workouts. This is totally normal. It is impossible to run like Carl Lewis when you're lifting like Arnold Schwarzenegger!

Women shouldn't be intimidated by the name of this phase. It is just as important for women as men to develop muscular strength. Don't worry—you won't end up muscle-bound. Just don't try to match weights with your significant other. Stay in a weight range that feels comfortable while making reasonable demands on your body.

The Power exercises require three sets. For set one, do 10 reps; set two, do 8 reps; and set three, do 6 reps. Set one will start out at a weight that is the same or slightly heavier than the weight you use during the endurance phase for the same exercise. Increase the weight for the second set so that you can complete the 8 reps with good form, but feel some burn by the end of the set. For set three, increase the weight as needed (if at all) so that the sixth and last rep takes everything you have.

During the Power phase, you will divide your exercises into two groups. On the first weight workout of the week, you will Power group A exercises (three sets of 10-8-6), while keeping the group B exercises the same as during the Endurance phase (two sets of 12 to 15). On the second weight workout of the week, you will Power group B exercises and keep group A at the level of the Endurance phase.

The Power exercises should be done in the same order as before. Note, however, that only the exercises indicated should be Powered. The other exercises are still done in two sets of 12

DAY 1		DAY 2	
Power	Lateral Pull-downs		Lateral Pull-downs
Power	Leg Extension		Leg Extension
Power	Leg Curls		Leg Curls
	Bench Press	**Power**	Bench Press
	Squats or Leg Press	**Power**	Squats or Leg Press
Power	Dumbbell Pullover		Dumbbell Pullover
	Bent Over Row		Bent Over Row
	Lunges		Lunges
	Side Lateral Raises		Side Lateral Raises
	Biceps	**Power**	Biceps
	Triceps	**Power**	Triceps
	Calf Raises		Calf Raises
	Sit-ups		Sit-ups
	Stretching		Stretching

to 15 reps. Also note that Day 1 has different exercises Powered than Day 2:

Note: Lateral raises and lunges are never Powered. Calf raises can be Powered if you wish. Some people suffer cramping if they Power the calf raises.

The Final Phase The final phase is called *Chisel*. This is where you take all the strength you have gained and hone it with repetitions that stimulate the speed of muscle contraction. In this phase, you will lighten the weight back down to the same as or slightly less than the weight used during the Endurance phase. You do two sets of 12 repetitions to the count of two on both the contraction and the relaxation.

This is a fast-paced action, very anaerobic in its feel. The weight should be chosen so that it feels light, yet becomes challenging at the end of the second set due to a mild lactic acid buildup. Failure starts to come from the speed of the move, not the load on the apparatus. Keep your form good, and make sure that there were still one or two reps left in you at the end of the second set.

7 Stretch It Good

Staying flexible is one way to reverse advancing age. Loss of strength, endurance, and flexibility awaits anyone who chooses an inactive lifestyle. However, if you remain active and choose a smart workout program that includes stretching, these same three criteria will remain at levels most people would consider impossible.

Several positive things happen when you are able to remain flexible. The first is that more flexibility equals less chance of injury. What good would an injury be for your health program?

Would nailing two boards to the front and back of your knees help you to be more flexible? Of course not! Stretching is like removing the boards. Joints like knees are able to move freely when the muscles that surround them are supple and flexible. If the fronts or backs of your legs are tight, then your knees are going to be held together more tightly. This puts added pressure on them. When you move, the friction on your knees is much greater than if you were looser. Become more flexible and the pressure is taken off the knees.

Think of yourself as a system of flowing currents. Flexibility keeps energy running smoothly through the entire system. Knotted muscles, stiff, shortened tendons, or joints that are held together tightly by inflexible muscles will all cause resistance in the body's energy flow.

As little as ten minutes of stretching a day will, over time, improve your flexibility tremendously.

Decreasing Your Aches and Pains If your neck is stiff, your attention is drawn all day long to that area. A lot of aches and pain that people feel as they get older can be chalked up to stiffness. It often goes away completely after going through a good stretching session. Increased flexibility may not cure every niggling problem you have, but it is the best insurance for not getting one in the first place.

Flexibility is not about being able to pull your feet behind your head when you're ninety-eight years old. Flexibility is about increasing your range of motion in all joints by loosening the muscles that hold those joints in place. It is also about increasing your ability to rotate your body from side to side by increasing flexibility in your spine, neck, and hips. Most motion appears linear at first glance but, if you think about it, even walking has rotational components to it. The only people who don't utilize this rotation are soldiers marching on display.

Having a greater range of motion makes any exercise easier. If you are tight, you fight against your own body. Part of your fatigue comes from muscles working against other muscles, each pulling in opposite directions. Got a tight hamstring? The quad will work harder to extend your leg out. Tight lats? Your shoulder will have to pull against it to get your arm fully over the water on the recovery portion of your swim stroke. Can't rotate your spine, neck, and hips? Every movement will be limited and every movement will use extra energy to pull against the tight axis of your body.

Flexibility and Performance If you have a broader range of motion with less resistance per stride during a marathon, it adds up to minutes off your overall time. The formula goes like this: One inch equals about $1/36$ of a stride. Over a four-hour marathon, one extra inch in your range of motion equates to 240 minutes divided by 36, or 6:40 minutes less in overall time. That is a significant amount, no matter what level you run at or aspire to. Time is saved simply because the body is not fighting itself for movement.

Go through a stretching program after your

> *It's better to stretch after a workout than before—that's when your muscles are warm. Stretching cold muscles is an invitation to injury.*

workout, when muscles are warmed up and take on the characteristics of soft, pliable plastic. Trying to stretch before a workout can cause your body actually to get tighter. Your muscles have a safety mechanism built in that will automatically cause them to snap tight to protect themselves against overstretching. When you are not warmed up, you can reach that defense stretch point very easily and end up causing your muscles to lock up and stay locked for a while.

Julie: Stretching I hate to admit it, but I don't really stretch. Over the years, I have done the next best thing by taking a long warm-up. However, now that my flexibility seems to be decreasing on a daily basis, I have been using yoga as a form of guided stretching. I lack the motivation to do it on my own, but I love the calm, focused environment of a yoga studio, especially with someone else leading me through the movements.

I would rather do two weekly sessions with a yoga instructor than struggle through fifteen minutes of stretching on my own. My favorite combo is to finish a weight workout or an aerobic workout and have a yoga class forty-five minutes to an hour after. I am warmed up before I go to the yoga, and mentally I am psyched.

Then I get the best of both worlds.

Mark: Start Slow I start every workout at a snail's pace. You would be shocked to see how slowly I start my runs. I'm usually going just slightly faster than a moderately brisk walk. I will keep this pace until my muscles begin to warm up and their motion increases without my even trying to make them do it. It may take fifteen to twenty minutes before my body really begins to loosen up. Eventually, my stride opens to its full, natural length.

I don't sprint when I get out of bed in the morning, so why would I sprint from the first step of my workout? Once I am finished with a workout, I go through my stretches.

Stretching to Prevent Injury *The most important time to stretch for injury prevention is when you are just starting to get into shape.* You are putting your body through a whole new set of physical stresses, and it is natural to have some soreness and stiffness. Once you get into shape, there will be less need to stretch, even though it should never be cut out completely.

Marathon Sitting Every profession has its peculiarities and possible injuries. If you spend long periods of time in a sitting position, your likelihood of having a tight lower back is significant. This includes everyone from taxi drivers and airplane pilots to executives and receptionists. Get up off the chair and stretch your psoas muscle. This muscle attaches to your lower vertebrae and can shorten during long periods of sitting. When you stand up, it is stretched—which can yank on your lower back, where it is attached, causing a lot of pain.

Arched-back push-ups and quad stretches work best to remedy the problem, along with generally working lower back rotation and, of course, doing regular exercise—which pumps blood and oxygen through an area that notoriously lacks both during sedentary periods.

How to Stretch The stretching suggested in this book is based on making stretches an extension of your workout. The end of the workout is the time to extend the natural process of muscle warming and loosening by doing stretches that mimic natural motions but in an exaggerated and isolated manner.

You can see from the following pictures that the larger muscles are stretched first, and that you switch from lateral to rotational stretches, working the entire body. The session should take five to twenty minutes, depending on how many times you make each movement.

Using this format will generally keep you from becoming even sorer from the stretches themselves. More extreme forms of stretching, like advanced yoga, can make you very sore. Stretching causes an inflammation response in your body just like any other damage that is caused by extreme movement. This program will minimize this response.

Never bounce a stretch. Move into the stretch gradually, holding it just for a second at the end of the action. If you are holding the stretch and the muscle feels like it is tightening up rather than loosening, back off. It's a sign the muscle is being overstretched. You are pushing what might be called the muscle's panic button.

Stretch after every workout that you think will make you sore or tight. Hard interval sessions, a long run, an outing that uses muscles you normally don't are all the perfect time to stretch. Everyday stretching is a matter of choice, but it's a *smart* choice.

The muscles in the body rely on a certain tension to bring you back to neutral once you reach your full extension. Take running, for example. Once you hit full stride, you have to bring your muscles back to neutral position. If you are too flexible, there won't be the natural snap from having just the right amount of tension in the muscles at full extension to bring it back quickly. Being Gumby can actually make you prone to injury just as being too tight can, although it is much more work to become too loose than it is to be too tight.

Julie: The Right Combination Right now, if you asked me the best workout combination, I would pick weights, yoga, and running. The weights and yoga together maintain my ability to run indefinitely. In yoga, you attain more of a dancer's posture. The muscles get an elongated, pretty shape, not a ripped athletic look. As I get older, I appreciate the softer lines your body gets through stretching.

Stretches

HAMSTRING ON BACK

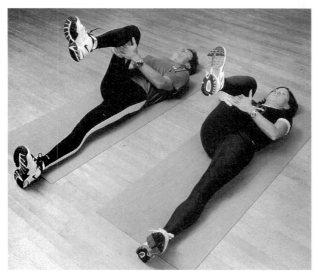

Beginning Position: Keeping one leg straight on the floor, raise the other with knee bent. Clasp the back of that leg with hands just behind your knee. Keep the other leg and back on the mat during the entire exercise.

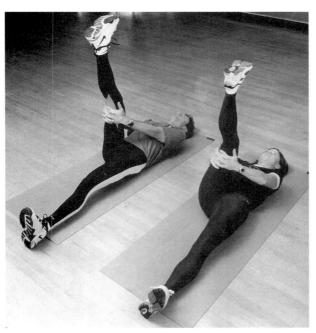

Ending Position: By arching your foot up, extend the bent leg until straight. Let this leg fall closer to the ground if necessary to extend the leg fully. With each repetition of the extension, try to pull the upper leg several inches closer to your chest.

QUADS ON SIDE

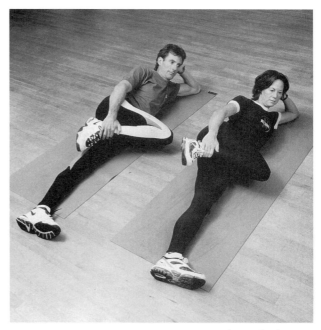

Beginning Position: Lying on your side with the bottom leg extended and the top knee bent, grasp the ankle of the bent leg and draw your knee close to your chest.

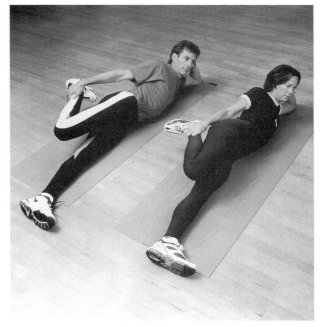

Ending Position: Pull the foot back until you feel a slight stretch in the quad. As you pull the leg back, push your hips forward to help add some stretch to the psoas muscle as well as the quad.

ROTATION: HIPS ON BACK

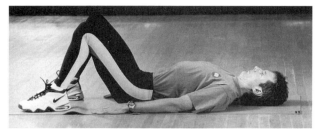

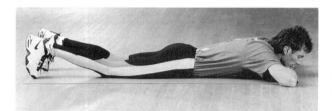

Beginning Position: Start with hands at your side, knees bent with feet on the ground.

Ending Position: Raise your hips off the ground, rotating them in as you contract your lower abs. A swivel movement happens as you raise your glutes and contract your abs.

ROTATION: HIPS ON STOMACH

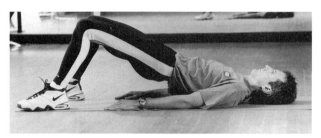

Beginning Position: This will move your lower back in the opposite direction as the previous stretch. Start lying on your stomach with your head straight, hands supporting your forehead. Tuck your toes in so they are raising your legs off of the floor just slightly.

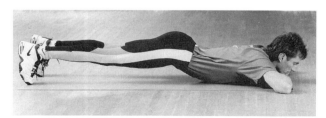

Ending Position: Arch your lower back and raise your hips off the mat. This will rotate your hips back instead of forward as the last stretch did.

PUSH-UP: LOWER BACK

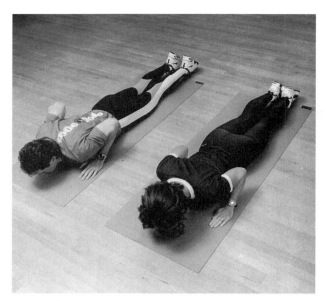

Beginning Position: Same as the previous stretch, but this time place your hands next to your mid-chest, ready to do a push-up.

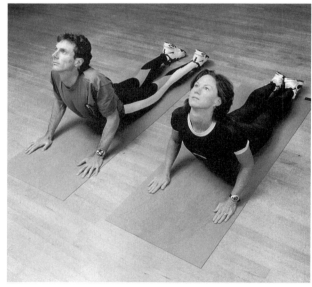

Ending Position: Keeping your hips on the mat, push up, arching your back and looking up toward the ceiling. Do this move in three positions: the first 5 to 10 reps with your head looking up, the next 5 to 10 reps looking over your left shoulder, then the final 5 to 10 reps looking over your right shoulder. Each time, come back to the neutral position with your head in the center.

ROTATION: CROSS LEGS AND DROP TO SIDE, WITH THREE HEAD POSITIONS

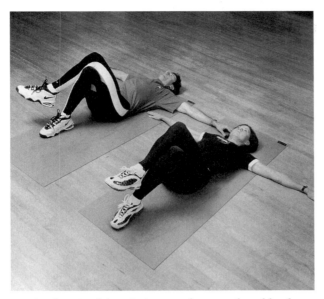

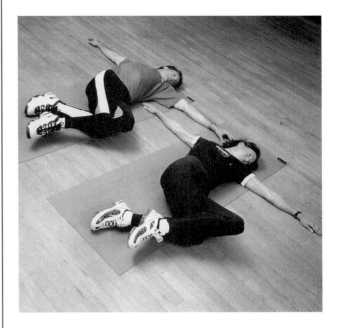

Beginning Position: Lying on the mat, bend both knees and cross one leg over the other. Let the top leg's lower part hang free. Arms are out straight.

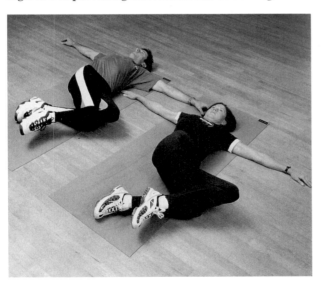

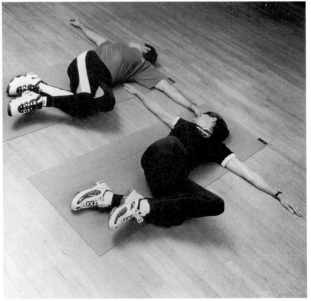

Ending Position: Drop both legs down toward the same side as the crossed-over leg. If you cross your right leg over the left one, lower both legs to the right. During the first 5 to 10 stretches, keep your head straight, looking toward the ceiling. Then do 5 to 10 reps where you turn your head to the opposite side as your dropped legs as you drop your legs. Bring your head back to neutral position when you raise your legs back up. Finally, do 5 to 10 reps and turn your head to the same side as the lowered legs.

ROTATION: BOOK ON FEET

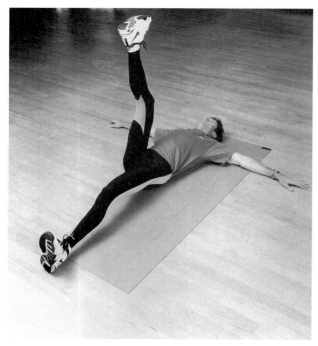

Beginning Position: Keep one leg flat on the mat. Extend the other leg up and pretend there is a book balanced on the bottom of that leg's foot.

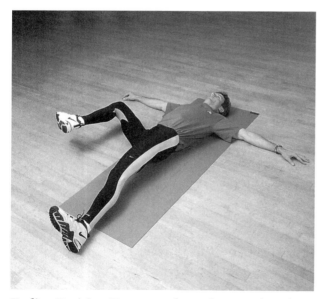

Ending Position: Drop your knee down and to the side, keeping your foot facing up, making sure that imaginary book doesn't fall off.

ROTATION: BOOK ON FEET ALL THE WAY TO STOMACH

Beginning Position: The starting position is the same as the previous stretch. However, this time the rotation is going to be in the opposite direction. Bring your knee down toward the floor, rotating your entire body toward the straight leg side.

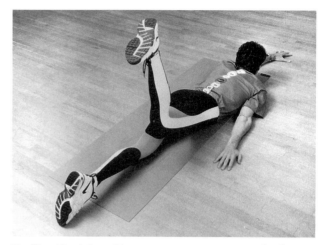

Ending Position: Keep rotating your entire body until you are on your stomach. Always keep the originally extended foot up toward the ceiling, again balancing the imaginary book on it.

ROTATION: HAMSTRINGS WITH THREE HAND POSITIONS

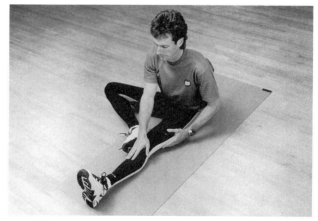

Beginning Position: One leg is extended and straight. The other is pulled in, with your foot placed close to the groin and the knee on the floor to the side. Put the hand that's on the straight leg side on the outside of that leg's quad. The other hand is placed on top of the quad.

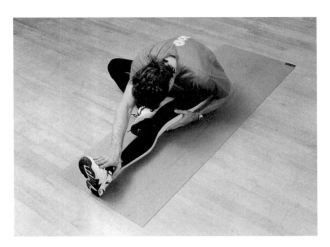

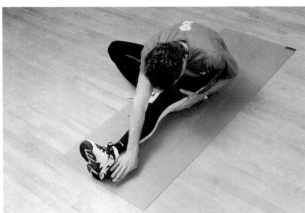

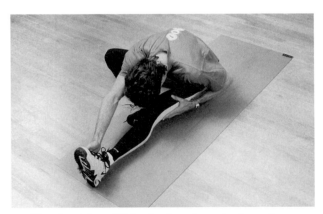

Ending Position: Slide the hand on the bent knee side toward your extended foot until a stretch is felt. Each time the move is repeated, try to extend the hands closer to the foot. Do 5 to 10 stretches with the hand sliding along the top of the leg, then 5 to 10 stretches sliding the hand toward the outside of the leg, and then 5 to 10 stretches sliding the hand along the inside of the leg. Each time, return to neutral position with the hand on the top of the quad.

WALKING UP TOE TOUCH

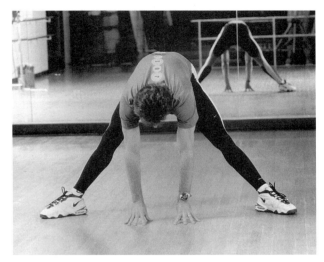

Beginning Position: Legs spread apart and knees straight. If possible, rest hands on floor. Point toes out.

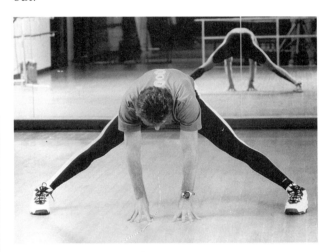

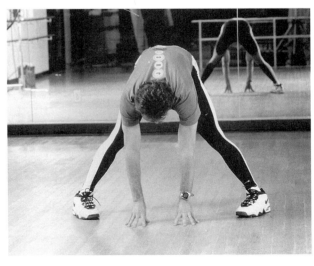

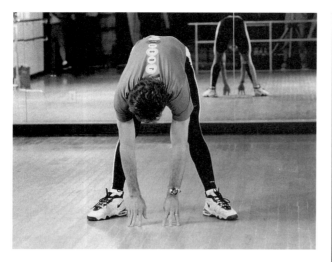

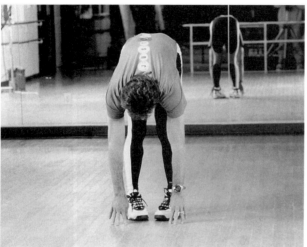

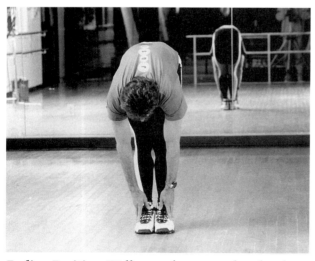

Ending Position: Walk your feet toward each other from this position, first turning the toes in, then turning the heels toward each other. Repeat this until the feet touch.

Extra Credit Those are the essentials of flexibility. If you want to try a few additional exercises, here are some samplers. Most are aimed at further increasing flexibility in the upper body.

TOWEL STRETCH

Using a small towel, grab one end with each hand and bring it behind your back just as you would do if you were going to dry your back off after a shower. Make sure that one arm is above the head and the other is below your head (as opposed to both at your side). Now work your hands closer together along the towel, trying to get both hands to touch. As the flexibility in your shoulders and arms increases over time, you will be able to clasp your hands together behind your back around the midback region.

STRAIGHT ARM STRETCH

Clasp your hands together behind your back. With elbows locked, raise your arms up as far as possible, trying to get them to be stretched out straight behind your back and parallel to the ground.

PECTORAL STRETCH

Find a wall or doorway. With your side to it, place one arm along the wall or doorframe parallel to the ground. Now twist your body, bringing the stretched arm as far behind the plane of your body as possible, stretching the pectorals and shoulder at the same time.

RIB CAGE STRETCH

Again using a wall or doorway, place both arms straight above your head at shoulder width on a wall or the top of a doorframe. Bend your torso forward, keeping your arms in place. Stretch as far as you can, again bringing the arms past the plane of your body, but this time stretch along the length of the body (instead of to the side as in the previous stretch).

Partner Stretches Sometimes stretching together is the only way you'll get any stretch at all. It can be enjoyable "together" time for a couple, as long as you don't push each other too hard. Gently help each other extend and hold the stretch. That's all.

With all of these stretches, make sure the one providing the stretch does not overstretch the muscle being worked. This is not a contest to see how flexible you can make your partner in ten minutes. Communication is the key. Bring the muscle into a *moderate* stretch, making sure you feel some stretch in the muscle but not one that is painful or extreme. Hold it for 5 seconds, then relax the stretch. Repeat 3 to 5 times.

TRICEPS

This is similar to the towel stretch, except that the arm is pulled back along the side of your head by your partner. Have him pull it back as you raise your arm up in a bent position.

PECTORALS

Clasp your partner's hands with her thumbs up behind her back, her arms straight, elbows not locked. Keep the arms parallel to the ground if they are flexible enough. Try to bring her hands closer and closer together with each hold of the stretch.

SHOULDER FLEXIBILITY

Use the same grip as the Pectoral Stretch, but hold your partner's palms facing the ground. Push the straight arms up behind his back, but do it gently. This is a good one for shoulder flexibility, but it is risky if there is any pain whatsoever in the shoulders of the person being stretched. So go easy.

LEGS

Just about every muscle group in the legs can be stretched with the help of a partner. Quads, hamstrings, glutes, and calves can all be done with two people. Simply help your partner into the stretch. Have him hold it like all the rest of the partner exercises for 3 to 5 seconds, then release the stretch. Repeat it 3 to 5 times, each time bringing a little more range of motion into the stretch if he is able.

One caution with hamstrings: This muscle can actually tighten up if the stretch is overdone. Go easy, especially if your partner already has tightness or cramping in the hamstring.

8 The Programs

I t's time to do it. All the mechanics of training have been laid out for you. The use of a heart-rate monitor to maximize your aerobic fitness has been described. The essentials of a strength program have been explained. And you have the concepts of flexibility with a lot of practical exercises that will keep your body running smoothly.

Now it's time to put it all into practice. What follows is a variety of sample training programs that will give you an idea of how to combine aerobic, anaerobic and strength training together.

Workout Programs The weekly schedules begin with a program that is designed to get your body into the rhythm of activity: Lifestyles Basic. It starts with a mixture of aer-

obic workouts, weights, and rest days. As you can see from the weekly minute totals, your activity will increase gradually over eighteen weeks. This particular program is for anyone who is just beginning to adopt an active lifestyle. This workout formula is excellent for both men and women.

By the end of this first schedule, you will be expending around 1,000 calories per week through exercise, which is about halfway to the optimal longevity expenditure of calories of 2,000 per week.

Next up is a schedule that will get you to that level: Lifestyles Advanced. This program picks up and builds on the fitness level attained through the Lifestyles Basic program. Most of you will be able to start at this level. By the end of the next eighteen weeks, your activity level will have you expending at least 2,000 calories per week, the optimal longevity formula!

Reading the Charts

Each eighteen-week schedule is divided into weekly sections. Below each day is the type of workout you will be doing. For aerobic workouts, the duration in time is listed in minutes—with the exception of swimming, which is listed in yards. Do the workouts with the heart rates that are specific for you as described by the MAHR formula in Chapter 5 (see page 52).

The weight workouts are abbreviated, with sets listed as 1×12, 2×15, etc. 1×12 is one set of 12 repetitions of each exercise. For the Power segments, refer back to Chapter 6 (see page 60) to see which exercises are Powered (one set of 10, one of 8, and one of 6), and which are still done like the Endurance phase (2×15).

Stay There or Keep Improving You can continue to cycle back through the Lifestyle Advanced schedule as many times as you like. When you are comfortable with this level of activity—or if you are already at this level of activity—you can move on to one of the sport programs that follow the Lifestyles Advanced section. You'll find the sprint triathlon and 10K schedules here.

We encourage you to work on a sport program. The added benefits to your fitness, your health, and your lifestyle are immense.

As with the Lifestyles programs, start with the Basic, then move on up to the Advanced ones. At this point, you will have the appropriate base of training for tackling either the Ironman triathlon schedules or the Marathon running program.

We wish you the best of luck.

WEEK	MONDAY Aerobic Activity	In Min.	TUESDAY 10 minutes Cardio/Weights	WEDNESDAY Rest/Optional Aerobic Activity	In Min.	THURSDAY Aerobic Activity	In Min.	FRIDAY Weights	SATURDAY Longer Aerobic Activity	In Min.	SUNDAY Rest/Optional Aerobic Activity	In Min.	TOTAL In Min.
1		20	ADA 1×12				20	ADA 1×12		20	OPT	20	60/80
2		25	ADA 1×12				25	ADA 1×12		25	OPT	20	75/95
3 RECOVERY		20	ADA 1×15				20	ADA 1×15		20	OPT	20	60/80
4		25	ADA 1×15				25	ADA 1×15		25	OPT	25	75/100
5		30	ADA 1×15				30	ADA 1×15		30	OPT	25	90/115
6 RECOVERY		25	END 2×12				25	END 2×12		25	OPT	25	75/100
7		30	END 2×12				30	END 2×12		30	OPT	30	90/120
8		35	END 2×12				35	END 2×12		35	OPT	30	105/135
9 RECOVERY		30	OFF				30	OFF		30	OPT	30	90/120
10		20	ADA 1×12				20	ADA 1×12		35	OPT	35	75/110
11		25	ADA 1×15		20		25	ADA 1×15		40	OPT	35	110/145
12 RECOVERY		20	END 2×12				20	END 2×12		35	OPT	35	75/110
13		25	END 2×12				25	END 2×12		40	OPT	40	90/130
14		30	END 2×15		25		30	END 2×15		45	OPT	40	130/170
15 RECOVERY		25	END 2×15				25	END 2×15		40	OPT	40	90/130
16		30	END 2×15				30	END 2×15		45	OPT	45	105/150
17		35	END 2×15		30		35	END 2×15		50	OPT	45	150/195
18 RECOVERY		30	OFF				30	OFF		45	OPT	45	105/150

Key

ADA=Adaptation, END=Endurance

Aerobic Activity: The choice is yours. Pick from a mix of any exercise that will enable you to raise your heart rate and hold it at that level for most of the workout. Outdoor options can include walking, running (or a combination of both), cycling, swimming, rowing, or hiking. If you like, head to the health club and use the treadmill, a stationary bike, stair-climber, or any other of the cardio equipment available at your gym.

Weights: As described in Chapter 6. It is important to do 10 to 15 minutes of light aerobic activity as a warm-up before doing the weights.

Longer Aerobic Activity: This is the perfect opportunity to choose an activity that is more nature-oriented. Use the fitness built on weekdays to get out in the wilds one day on the weekends. Or, if you still choose an activity like cycling, make this one a mountain-bike ride instead of on the roads. You may find that 50 to 60 minutes is not enough. Let it rip!

WEEK	MONDAY Aerobic Activity	In Min.	TUESDAY 10 minutes Cardio/Weights	WEDNESDAY Aerobic Activity	In Min.	THURSDAY Aerobic Activity	In Min.	FRIDAY Weights	SATURDAY Longer Aerobic Activity	In Min.	SUNDAY Rest/Optional Aerobic Activity	In Min.	TOTAL In Min.
1		30	ADA 1×12				30	ADA 1×12		250	OPT	40	140/180
2		35	ADA 1×12		35		35	ADA 1×15		55	OPT	40	160/200
3 RECOVERY		30	ADA 1×15		OFF		30	ADA 1×15		50	OPT	40	110/150
4		35	END 2×12		35		35	END 2×12		55	OPT	45	160/205
5		40	END 2×12		40		40	END 2×12		60	OPT	45	160/225
6 RECOVERY		35	END 2×15		OFF		35	END 2×15		55	OPT	45	160/170
7		40	END 2×15		35		40	END 2×15		60	OPT	50	175/225
8		45	END 2×15		40		45	END 2×15		70	OPT	50	200/250
9 RECOVERY		40	END 2×15		OFF		40	END 2×15		60	OPT	50	140/190
10		45	END 2×15		35		45	END 2×15		70	OPT	60	195/255
11		50	END 2×15		40		50	END 2×15		80	OPT	60	220/280
12 RECOVERY		35	POW A		30		35	POW B		70	OPT	60	170/230
13		45	POW A		35		45	POW B		80	OPT	70	205/275
14		50	POW A		40		50	POW B		90	OPT	70	230/300
15 RECOVERY		35	POW A		30		35	POW B		80	OPT	70	180/250
16		45	CHI 2×12		35		45	CHI 2×12		90	OPT	80	215/295
17		50	CHI 2×12		40		50	CHI 2×12		100	OPT	80	240/320
18 RECOVERY		30	OFF		30		30	OFF		60	OPT	80	150/230

Key

ADA=Adaptation, **END**=Endurance, **POW**=Power, **CHI**=Chisel

Aerobic Activity: The choice is yours. Pick from a mix of any exercise that will enable you to raise your heart rate and hold it at that level for most of the workout. Outdoor options can include walking, running (or a combination of both), cycling, swimming, rowing, or hiking. If you like, head to the health club and use the treadmill, a stationary bike, stair-climber, or any other of the cardio equipment available at your gym.

Weights: As described in Chapter 6. It is important to do 10 to 15 minutes of light aerobic activity as a warm-up before doing the weights.

Longer Aerobic Activity: This is the perfect opportunity to choose an activity that is more nature-oriented. Use the fitness built on weekdays to get out in the wilds one day on the weekends. Or, if you still choose an activity like cycling, make this one a mountain-bike ride instead of on the roads. You may find that 50 to 60 minutes is not enough. Let it rip!

10K Basic

WEEK	MONDAY	TUESDAY	WEDNESDAY	THURSDAY	In Min.	FRIDAY	SATURDAY	In Min.	SATURDAY	SUNDAY	In Min.	TOTAL
	Run Easy Recovery in Min.	Warm-up/ Weights	Run Moderate Aerobic/ Endurance in Min.	Run High Aerobic or Speed	In Min.	Rest/ Endurance	Run Moderate Aerobic	In Min.	Warm-up/ Weights	Run Endurance	In Min.	In Min.
1	30	OFF	30		40	OFF		30	OFF		40	170
2	30	ADA 1×12	40		30	OFF		30	ADA 1×12		50	180
3	30	ADA 1×12	45		35	OFF		25	ADA 1×15		60	195
4 RECOVERY	30	ADA 1×15	45		30	OFF	10×10SEC. SURGES	20	OFF	10K RACE	60	185
5	30	END 2×12	40		35	OFF		35	END 2×12		70	210
6	30	END 2×12	45		40	OFF		30	END 2×12		80	225
7 RECOVERY	40	END 2×15	40		35	OFF		25	END 2×15		60	200
8	40	END 2×15	50		40	OFF		30	END 2×15		90	250
9	40	END 2×15	60		35	OFF	10×10SEC. SURGES	20	OFF	10 MILE RACE	100	255
10 BEGIN SPEED	35	END 2×15	45	8×400, 4×100	45	OFF		35	END 2×15		80	240
11	35	POW A	45	1×1MI., 1×800, 4×400	50	OFF		40	POW B		90	260
12	35	POW A	45	3×5MIN. HILLS	50	OFF		45	POW B		100	275
13 RECOVERY	35	POW A	35	8×400, 4×100	45	OFF		25	POW B		70	210
14 LONGEST RUN	40	CHI 2×12	50	3×3MIN., 1×9MIN., 3×1MIN. HILLS	60	OFF		40	CHI 2×12		100	290
15 BEGIN TAPER	30	CHI 2×12	40	2×1000, 4×400	45	OFF		40	CHI 2×12		80	235
16	30	OFF	35	5×90SEC., 5×30SEC. HILLS	45	OFF	10×10SEC. SURGES	20	OFF	5K RACE	30	160
17	30	OFF	35	2×1MI. STRAIGHTS & CURVES	40	OFF		30	OFF		45	180
18	30	OFF	30	EASY	20	OFF	10×10SEC. SURGES	20	OFF	10K RACE	60	160

Key

ADA=Adaptation, **END**=Endurance, **POW**=Power, **CHI**=Chisel

Easy Recovery: These are for recovery at heart rates at the very low end of aerobic ranges, approximately 20 to 30 beats below your Maximum Aerobic Heart Rate (MAHR).

Moderate Aerobic: Runs keeping your heart rate from 20 to 30 beats below up to 5 beats below your MAHR.

High Aerobic: The bulk of the workout, once you're warmed up, is held within 10 beats of your MAHR.

Endurance: Heart rates from 20 to 30 below your MAHR up to it.

Speed: Heart rates above your MAHR. Warm up for 10 to 15 minutes, gradually increasing speed and heart rate. Then, for each interval, continue to increase your heart rate, trying to get it above your MAHR on the first one and increasing it a beat or two for each one after that. The rest between should be enough to let your heart rate drop at least as low as your MAHR if not 20 to 30 below it. *Straights and curves:* Run the straight sections of a running track fast, then jog more slowly around the curves.

WEEK	MONDAY Run Easy Recovery in Min.	TUESDAY Warm-up/Weights	WEDNESDAY Run Moderate Aerobic/Endurance in Min.	THURSDAY Run High Aerobic or Speed	In Min.	FRIDAY Rest/Run Endurance in Min.	SATURDAY Run Moderate Aerobic	In Min.	SATURDAY Warm-up/Weights	SUNDAY Run Endurance	In Min.	TOTAL In Min.
1	30	OFF	30		40	OFF		30	OFF		50	180
2	30	ADA 1×12	40		30	OFF		30	ADA 1×12		60	190
3	30	ADA 1×12	45		35	60		25	ADA 1×15		70	265
4 RECOVERY	30	ADA 1×15	45		30	OFF	10×10SEC. SURGES	30	OFF	10K RACE	40	175
5	30	END 2×12	40		35	OFF		35	END 2×12		70	210
6	30	END 2×12	40		40	70		30	END 2×12		80	290
7 RECOVERY	40	END 2×15	40		35	OFF		25	END 2×15		70	210
8	40	END 2×15	50		45	80		30	END 2×15		90	335
9	40	END 2×15	50		40	OFF	10×10SEC. SURGES	30	OFF	10 MILE RACE	65	225
10 BEGIN SPEED	35	END 2×15	50	8×400, 8×100	45	OFF		35	END 2×15		80	245
11	40	POW A	70	1×1MI. 2×800, 4×400, 6×100	50	OFF		40	POW B		90	290
12	40	POW A	50	4×5MIN. HILLS	50	OFF		45	POW B		90	275
13 RECOVERY	40	POW A	60	8×400, 8×100	45	OFF		25	POW B		70	240
14 LONGEST RUN	40	CHI 2×12	30	3×4MIN., 1×9MIN., 3×3MIN. HILLS	60	OFF		45	CHI 2×12		100	275
15 BEGIN TAPER	30	CHI 2×12	50	3×1000, 4×400, 8×100	45	OFF		45	CHI 2×12		80	250
16	30	OFF	60	5×90SEC., 5×30SEC. HILLS	45	OFF	10×10SEC. SURGES	20	OFF	5K RACE	20	175
17	30	OFF	45	2×1MI. STRAIGHTS & CURVES		OFF		30	OFF		45	150
18	30	OFF	35	OFF		EASY 25	10×10SEC. SURGES	20	OFF	10K RACE	40	150

Key

ADA=Adaptation, **END**=Endurance, **POW**=Power, **CHI**=Chisel

Easy Recovery: These are for recovery at heart rates at the very low end of aerobic ranges, approximately 20 to 30 beats below your Maximum Aerobic Heart Rate (MAHR).

Moderate Aerobic: Runs keeping your heart rate from 20 to 30 beats below up to a heart rate of 5 beats below your MAHR.

High Aerobic: For the bulk of the workout, once warmed up, you keep your heart rate within 10 beats of your MAHR.

Endurance: Heart rates from 20 to 30 below your MAHR up to it.

Speed: Heart rates above your MAHR. Warm up for 10 to 15 minutes, gradually increasing speed and heart rate. Then, for each interval, continue to increase your heart rate, trying to get it above your MAHR on the first one and increasing it a beat or two for each one after that. The rest between should be enough to let your heart rate drop at least as low as your MAHR if not 20 to 30 below it. *Straights and curves:* Run the straight sections of a running track fast, then jog more slowly around the curves.

WEEK TO RACE	WEEK	MONDAY	TUESDAY	WEDNESDAY	THURSDAY	FRIDAY	SATURDAY	SUNDAY
18	1	OFF	OFF	OFF	OFF	OFF	OFF	
17	2	OFF	ADA	OFF	OFF	ADA	OFF	
16	3	OFF	ADA	OFF	OFF	ADA	OFF	
15	4 RECOVERY	OFF	ADA	OFF	OFF	OFF	OFF	10K RACE
14	5	OFF	END	OFF	OFF	END	OFF	
13	6	OFF	END	OFF	OFF	END	OFF	
12	7 RECOVERY	OFF	END	OFF	OFF	END	OFF	
11	8	OFF	END	OFF	OFF	END	OFF	
10	9	OFF	END	OFF	OFF	OFF	OFF	10 MILE RACE
9	10 BEGIN SPEED	OFF	END	OFF	OFF	END	OFF	
8	11	OFF	POW	OFF	OFF	POW	OFF	
7	12	OFF	POW	OFF	OFF	POW	OFF	
6	13 RECOVERY	OFF	POW	OFF	OFF	POW	OFF	
5	14 LONGEST RUN	OFF	CHI	OFF	OFF	CHI	OFF	
4	15 BEGIN TAPER	OFF	CHI	OFF	OFF	CHI	OFF	
3	16	OFF	OFF	OFF	OFF	OFF	OFF	5K RACE
2	17	OFF	OFF	OFF	OFF	OFF	OFF	
1	18	OFF	OFF	OFF	OFF	OFF	OFF	10K RACE

Key

ADA=Adaptation, **END**=Endurance, **POW**=Power, **CHI**=Chisel

Adaptation: 1 set of 12 to 15 reps. (Lift on a count of two, lower on a count of four.)

Endurance: 2 sets of 12 to 15 reps.

Power: Tuesday: Power group A exercises (1 × 10, 1 × 8, 1 × 6), the rest as in Endurance.
Friday: Power group B exercises (1 × 10, 1 × 8, 1 × 6), the rest as in Endurance.

Chisel: 2 sets of 12 reps. (Lift and lower on a count of two.)

Olympic Distance Triathlon Basic

WEEK	MONDAY	TUESDAY	WEDNESDAY	THURSDAY	FRIDAY	SATURDAY	SUNDAY	TOTAL
SWIM	Moderate Aerobic in Yards	Rest	Endurance in Yards	Rest	High Aerobic or Speed in Yards	Off or Easy in Yards	Rest or Race in Yards	In Yards
1 EASY	2000	OFF	2500	OFF	2500	OFF	OFF	7000
2	2000	OFF	3000	OFF	2500	OFF	OFF	7500
3	2000	OFF	3500	OFF	3000	OFF	OFF	8500
4 RECOVERY	2500	OFF	3000	OFF	OFF	10×10SEC. SURGES 500	OLYMPIC DISTANCE 1500	7500
5	1000	OFF	2500	OFF	2500	OFF	OFF	6000
6	2500	OFF	4000	OFF	3000	OFF	OFF	9500
7 RECOVERY	2000	OFF	3000	OFF	2500	OFF	OFF	7500
8	3000	OFF	3500	OFF	2500	OFF	OFF	9000
9	2500	OFF	3000	OFF	OFF	10×10SEC. SURGES 500	OLYMPIC DISTANCE 1500	7500
10 BEGIN SPEED	1000	OFF	3500	OFF	2500	OFF	OFF	7000
11	1500	OFF	3500	OFF	3000	OFF	OFF	8000
12	3000	OFF	4000	OFF	2500	OFF	OFF	9500
13 RECOVERY	2000	OFF	3500	OFF	2500	OFF	OFF	8000
14 LONGEST WEEK	3500	OFF	4000	OFF	3000	OFF	OFF	10500
15 BEGIN TAPER	2500	OFF	3500	OFF	2500	OFF	OFF	8500
16	2000	OFF	3000	OFF	OFF	10×10SEC. SURGES 500	SPRING TRIATHLON 500	6000
17	2000	OFF	3000	OFF	2500	OFF	OFF	7500
18	1500	OFF	2000	OFF	OFF	10×10SEC. SURGES 500	OLYMPIC DISTANCE 1500	5500

Key

Easy Recovery: These are for recovery at heart rates at the very low end of aerobic ranges, approximately 20 to 30 beats below your Maximum Aerobic Heart Rate (MAHR).

Moderate Aerobic: Swims keeping your heart rate from 20 to 30 beats below up to a heart rate of 5 beats below your MAHR.

High Aerobic: For the bulk of the workout, once warmed up, you keep your heart rate within 10 beats of your MAHR.

Endurance: Heart rates from 20 to 30 below your MAHR up to it.

Speed: Heart rates above your MAHR. Warm up to 10 to 15 minutes, gradually increasing speed and heart rate. Then, for each interval, continue to increase your heart rate, trying to get it above your MAHR on the first one and increasing it a beat or two for each one after that. The rest between should be enough to let your heart rate drop at least as low as your MAHR if not 20 to 30 below.

Olympic Distance Triathlon Basic

WEEK	MONDAY	TUESDAY	WEDNESDAY	THURSDAY	In Min.	FRIDAY	SATURDAY	SUNDAY	In Min.	TOTAL
BIKE	Rest	Moderate Aerobic/ Endurance In Min.	Rest	High Aerobic or Speed	In Min.	Rest	Endurance In Min.	Rest or Race	In Min.	In Min.
1 EASY	OFF	60	OFF		60	OFF	90	OFF		210
2	OFF	60	OFF		60	OFF	120	OFF		240
3	OFF	60	OFF		90	OFF	120	OFF		270
4 RECOVERY	OFF	60	OFF		45	OFF	10×10SEC. SURGES 30	OLYMPIC DISTANCE	90	225
5	OFF	60	OFF		75	OFF	120	OFF		255
6	OFF	60	OFF		90	OFF	150	OFF		300
7 RECOVERY	OFF	60	OFF		60	OFF	90	OFF		210
8	OFF	60	OFF		90	OFF	150	OFF		300
9	OFF	60	OFF		45	OFF	10×10SEC. SURGES 30	OLYMPIC DISTANCE	90	225
10 BEGIN SPEED	OFF	60	OFF	10×1MIN.	60	OFF	150	OFF		270
11	OFF	60	OFF	1×5MIN., 5×2MIN.	60	OFF	180	OFF		300
12	OFF	90	OFF	3×5MIN. HILLS	60	OFF	180	OFF		330
13 RECOVERY	OFF	60	OFF	10×90SEC.	60	OFF	120	OFF		240
14 LONGEST WEEK	OFF	90	OFF	1×20MIN. HILLS OR TIME TRIAL	60	OFF	210	OFF		350
15 BEGIN TAPER	OFF	90	OFF	3×3MIN., 2×2MIN., 4×1MIN.	60	OFF	150	OFF		300
16	OFF	90	OFF	EASY	60	OFF	10×10 SEC. SURGES 30	SPRINT TRIATHLON	30	210
17	OFF	75	OFF	1×5MIN., 4×1MIN.	60	OFF	90	OFF		225
18	OFF	45	OFF	EASY	45	OFF	10×10SEC. SURGES 30	OLYMPIC DISTANCE	90	210

Key

Easy Recovery: These are for recovery at heart rates at the very low end of aerobhic ranges, approximately 20 to 30 beats below your Maximum Aerobic Heart Rate (MAHR).

Moderate Aerobic: Bike rides keeping your heart rate from 20 to 30 beats below up to a heart rate of 5 beats below your MAHR.

High Aerobic: For the bulk of the workout, once warmed up, you keep your heart rate within 10 beats of your MAHR.

Endurance: Heart rates from 20 to 30 below your MAHR up to it.

Speed: Heart rates above your MAHR. Warm up to 10 to 15 minutes, gradually increasing speed and heart rate. Then, for each interval, continue to increase your heart rate, trying to get it above your MAHR on the first one and increasing it a beat or two for each one after that. The rest between should be enough to let your heart rate drop at least as low as your MAHR if not 20 to 30 below it.

WEEK	MONDAY	TUESDAY	WEDNESDAY	THURSDAY	In Min.	FRIDAY	SATURDAY	In Min.	SUNDAY	In Min.	TOTAL In Min.
RUN	Easy Recovery in Min.	Rest/Easy	Moderate Aerobic/Endurance in Min.	High Aerobic or Speed		Rest/Endurance	Moderate Aerobic		Endurance		
1 EASY	30	OFF	30		40	OFF	OFF			40	110
2	30	OFF	40		30	OFF	OFF			45	145
3	30	OFF	50	OFF		OFF	AFTER BIKE	25		50	155
4 RECOVERY	30	OFF	35	OFF		OFF	10×10SEC. SURGES	20	OLYMPIC DISTANCE	60	145
5	30	OFF	OFF		40	OFF	OFF			60	130
6	30	OFF	45	OFF		OFF	AFTER BIKE	30		75	180
7 RECOVERY	40	OFF	OFF		35	OFF	OFF			60	135
8	40	OFF	50		40	OFF	AFTER BIKE	30		70	230
9	40	OFF	35	OFF		OFF	10×10SEC. SURGES	20	OLYMPIC DISTANCE	60	155
10 BEGIN SPEED	35	OFF	OFF	8×400	45	OFF	OFF			70	150
11	35	OFF	OFF	1×1MI., 1×800, 4×400	50	OFF	OFF			75	160
12	45	OFF	OFF	3×5MIN. HILLS	50	OFF	AFTER BIKE	35		80	210
13 RECOVERY	35	OFF	OFF	8×400, 4×100	45	OFF	OFF			60	140
14 LONGEST WEEK	40	OFF	35	1×9MIN, 3×1MIN. HILLS	50	OFF	AFTER BIKE	45		90	260
15 BEGIN TAPER	30	OFF	OFF	2×1000, 4×400	45	OFF	AFTER BIKE	40		60	175
16	35	OFF	OFF	5×90SEC., 5×30SEC. HILLS	40	OFF	10×10SEC. SURGES	20	SPRINT TRIATHLON	30	125
17	30	OFF	OFF	2×1MI. STRAIGHTS & CURVES	40	OFF	OFF			45	115
18	30	OFF	30	OFF		OFF	10×10SEC. SURGES	20	OLYMPIC DISTANCE	60	140

Key

Easy Recovery: These are for recovery at heart rates at the very low end of aerobic ranges, approximately 20 to 30 beats below your Maximum Aerobic Heart Rate (MAHR).

Moderate Aerobic: Runs keeping your heart rate from 20 to 30 beats below up to 5 beats below your MAHR.

High Aerobic: The bulk of the workout, once warmed up, is held within 10 beats of your MAHR.

Endurance: Heart rates from 20 to 30 below your MAHR up to it.

Speed: Heart rates above your MAHR. Warm up for 10 to 15 minutes, gradually increasing speed and heart rate. Then, for each interval, continue to increase your heart rate, trying to get it above your MAHR on the first one and increasing it a beat or two for each one after that. The rest between should be enough to let your heart rate drop at least as low as your MAHR, if not 20 to 30 below it. *Straights and curves:* Run the straight sections of a running track fast, then jog more slowly around the curves.

WEEK	MONDAY	TUESDAY	WEDNESDAY	THURSDAY	FRIDAY	SATURDAY	SUNDAY	TOTAL
SWIM	Moderate Aerobic in Yards	Rest	Endurance in Yards	Rest	High Aerobic or Speed in Yards	Off or Easy (In Yards)	Rest or Race (In Yards)	In Yards
1 EASY	2500	OFF	3000	OFF	2500	OFF	OFF	8000
2	3000	OFF	3500	OFF	2500	OFF	EASY 2000	11000
3	3000	OFF	4000	OFF	3000	OFF	EASY 1500	11500
4 RECOVERY	2500	OFF	3000	OFF	OFF	10×10SEC. SURGES 500	OLYMPIC DISTANCE 1500	7500
5	1000	OFF	2500	OFF	3000	OFF	OFF	6500
6	3500	OFF	4000	OFF	3000	OFF	1500	12000
7 RECOVERY	2500	OFF	3500	OFF	2500	OFF	OFF	8500
8	3000	OFF	4000	OFF	2500	OFF	1500	11000
9	2500	OFF	3000	OFF	OFF	10×10 SEC. SURGES 500	OLYMPIC DISTANCE 1500	7500
10 BEGIN SPEED	1500	OFF	3500	OFF	2500	OFF	1500	9000
11	1500	OFF	4000	OFF	3000	OFF	OFF	8500
12	3000	OFF	4500	OFF	3000	OFF	2000	12500
13 RECOVERY	2000	OFF	3500	OFF	2500	OFF	OFF	8000
14 LONGEST WEEK	3500	OFF	4500	OFF	3500	OFF	2000	13500
15 BEGIN TAPER	2500	OFF	3500	OFF	3000	OFF	1500	10500
16	2000	OFF	3000	OFF	OFF	10×10SEC. SURGES 500	SPRING TRIATHLON 500	6000
17	2000	OFF	3000	OFF	2500	OFF	OFF	7500
18	2500	OFF	2000	OFF	OFF	10×10SEC. SURGES 500	OLYMPIC DISTANCE 1500	6500

Key

Easy Recovery: These are for recovery at heart rates at the very low end of aerobic ranges, approximately 20 to 30 beats below your Maximum Aerobic Heart Rate (MAHR).

Moderate Aerobic: Swims keeping your heart rate from 20 to 30 beats below up to a heart rate of 5 beats below your MAHR.

High Aerobic: For the bulk of the workout, once warmed up, you keep your heart rate within 10 beats of your MAHR.

Endurance: Heart rates from 20 to 30 below your MAHR up to it.

Speed: Heart rates above your MAHR. Warm up for 10 to 15 minutes, gradually increasing speed and heart rate. Then, for each interval, continue to increase your heart rate, trying to get it above your MAHR on the first one and increasing it a beat or two for each one after that. The rest between should be enough to let your heart rate drop at least as low as your MAHR, if not 20 to 30 below it.

Olympic Distance Triathlon
Advanced

WEEK	MONDAY	TUESDAY	WEDNESDAY	THURSDAY	In Min.	FRIDAY	SATURDAY	In Min.	SUNDAY	In Min.	TOTAL
BIKE	Rest	Moderate Aerobic/ Endurance in Min.	Rest	High Aerobic or Speed	In Min.	Rest	Endurance	In Min.	Rest or Race	In Min.	In Min.
1 EASY	OFF	60	OFF		60	OFF		120	OFF		240
2	OFF	60	OFF		60	OFF		150	EASY	60	330
3	OFF	90	OFF		60	OFF		180	OFF		330
4 RECOVERY	OFF	75	OFF		45	OFF	10×10SEC. SURGES	30	OLYMPIC DISTANCE	75	225
5	OFF	60	OFF		60	OFF		150		60	330
6	OFF	60	OFF		60	OFF		180		60	360
7 RECOVERY	OFF	60	OFF		60	OFF		150	OFF		270
8	OFF	120	OFF		90	OFF		180	OFF		390
9	OFF	75	OFF		45	OFF	10×10SEC. SURGES	30	OLYMPIC DISTANCE	75	225
10 BEGIN SPEED	OFF	60	OFF	10×1 MIN.	60	OFF		180	OFF		300
11	OFF	90	OFF	1×5MIN., 5×2MIN.	60	OFF		210		60	420
12	OFF	90	OFF	3×5MIN. HILLS	60	OFF		240		60	450
13 RECOVERY	OFF	60	OFF	10×2MIN.	60	OFF		180	OFF		300
14 LONGEST WEEK	OFF	90	OFF	1×20MIN. HILLS OR TIME TRIAL	60	OFF		270		60	480
15 BEGIN TAPER	OFF	90	OFF	3×3MIN., 2×2MIN., 4×1MIN.	60	OFF		180	OFF		330
16	OFF	120	OFF	EASY	60	OFF	10×10SEC. SURGES	30	SPRINT TRIATHLON	25	235
17	OFF	75	OFF	1×5MIN., 4×2MIN.	60	OFF		90	OFF		225
18	OFF	60	OFF	EASY	45	OFF	10×10SEC. SURGES	30	OLYMPIC DISTANCE	75	210

Key

Easy Recovery: These are for recovery at heart rates at the very low end of aerobic ranges, approximately 20 to 30 beats below your Maximum Aerobic Heart Rate (MAHR).

Moderate Aerobic: Bike rides keeping your heart rate from 20 to 30 beats below up to a heart rate of 5 beats below your MAHR.

High Aerobic: For the bulk of the workout, once warmed up, you keep your heart rate within 10 beats of your MAHR.

Endurance: Heart rates from 20 to 30 below your MAHR up to it.

Speed: Heart rates above your MAHR. Warm up for 10 to 15 minutes, gradually increasing speed and heart rate. Then, for each interval, continue to increase your heart rate, trying to get it above your MAHR on the first one and increasing it a beat or two for each one after that. The rest between should be enough to let your heart rate drop at least as low as your MAHR, if not 20 to 30 below it.

WEEK	MONDAY	TUESDAY	WEDNESDAY	THURSDAY		FRIDAY	SATURDAY		SUNDAY		TOTAL
RUN	Easy Recovery in Min.	Rest/Easy	Moderate Aerobic/Endurance in Min.	High Aerobic or Speed	In Min.	Rest/Endurance	Moderate Aerobic	In Min.	Endurance	In Min.	In Min.
1 EASY	30	OFF	30		40	OFF	OFF			50	120
2	30	OFF	40		30	OFF	OFF			60	160
3	30	OFF	50	OFF OFF		OFF	AFTER BIKE	25		55	160
4 RECOVERY	30	OFF	35	OFF		OFF	10×10SEC. SURGES	20	OLYMPIC DISTANCE	45	130
5	30	OFF	OFF		40	OFF	OFF			70	140
6	30	OFF	45	OFF		OFF	AFTER BIKE	30		90	195
7 RECOVERY	40	OFF	OFF		35	OFF	OFF			70	145
8	40	OFF	50		40	OFF	AFTER BIKE	30		75	235
9	40	OFF	35	OFF		OFF	10×10SEC. SURGES	20	OLYMPIC DISTANCE	45	140
10 BEGIN SPEED	35	OFF	OFF	8×400, 8×100	45	OFF	OFF			75	155
11	35	OFF	OFF	1×1MI., 2×800, 4×400, 6×100	50	OFF	OFF			90	175
12	45	OFF	OFF	4×5MIN. HILLS	50	OFF	AFTER BIKE	35		100	230
13 RECOVERY	35	OFF	OFF	8×400, 8×100	45	OFF	OFF			70	150
14 LONGEST WEEK	40	OFF	45	1×9MIN., 3×3MIN. HILLS	50	OFF	AFTER BIKE	45		100	280
15 BEGIN TAPER	30	OFF	OFF	3×1000, 4×400, 8×100	45	OFF	AFTER BIKE	40		75	190
16	35	OFF	OFF	5×90SEC., 5×30SEC. HILLS	40	OFF	10×10SEC. SURGES	20	SPRINT TRIATHLON	30	125
17	30	OFF	OFF	2×1MI. STRAIGHTS & CURVES	40	OFF	OFF			50	120
18	35	OFF	30	OFF		OFF	10×10SEC. SURGES	20	OLYMPIC DISTANCE	60	145

Key

Easy Recovery: These are for recovery at heart rates at the very low end of aerobic ranges, approximately 20 to 30 beats below your Maximum Aerobic Heart Rate (MAHR).

Moderate Aerobic: Runs keeping your heart rate from 20 to 30 beats below up to a heart rate of 5 beats below your MAHR.

High Aerobic: The bulk of the workout, once warmed up, is held within 10 beats of your MAHR.

Endurance: Heart rates from 20 to 30 below your MAHR up to it.

Speed: Heart rates above your MAHR. Warm up for 10 to 15 minutes, gradually increasing speed and heart rate. Then, for each interval, continue to increase your heart rate, trying to get it above your MAHR on the first one and increasing it a beat or two for each one after that. The rest between should be enough to let your heart rate drop at least as low as your MAHR, if not 20 to 30 below it. *Straights and curves:* Run the straight sections of a running track fast, then jog more slowly around the curves.

Olympic Distance Triathlon Weights

WEEK TO RACE	WEEK	MONDAY	TUESDAY	WEDNESDAY	THURSDAY	FRIDAY	SATURDAY	SUNDAY
18	1	OFF	OFF	OFF	OFF	OFF	OFF	
17	2	OFF	ADA 1×12	OFF	OFF	ADA 1×12	OFF	
16	3	OFF	ADA 1×12	OFF	OFF	ADA 1×15	OFF	
15	4 RECOVERY	OFF	ADA 1×15	OFF	OFF	OFF	OFF	OLYMPIC DISTANCE
14	5	OFF	END 2×12	OFF	OFF	END 2×12	OFF	
13	6	OFF	END 2×12	OFF	OFF	END 2×12	OFF	
12	7 RECOVERY	OFF	END 2×15	OFF	OFF	END 2×15	OFF	
11	8	OFF	END 2×15	OFF	OFF	END 2×15	OFF	
10	9	OFF	END 2×15	OFF	OFF	OFF	OFF	OLYMPIC DISTANCE
9	10 BEGIN SPEED	OFF	END 2×15	OFF	OFF	END 2×15	OFF	
8	11	OFF	POW A	OFF	OFF	POW B	OFF	
7	12	OFF	POW A	OFF	OFF	POW B	OFF	
6	13 RECOVERY	OFF	POW A	OFF	OFF	POW B	OFF	
5	14 LONGEST RUN	OFF	CHI 2×12	OFF	OFF	CHI 2×12	OFF	
4	15 BEGIN TAPER	OFF	CHI 2×12	OFF	OFF	CHI 2×12	OFF	
3	16	OFF	OFF	OFF	OFF	OFF	OFF	SPRINT TRIATHLON
2	17	OFF	OFF	OFF	OFF	OFF	OFF	
1	18	OFF	OFF	OFF	OFF	OFF	OFF	OLYMPIC DISTANCE

Key

ADA=Adaptation, **END**=Endurance, **POW**=Power, **CHI**=Chisel

Adaptation: 1 set of 12 to 15 reps. (Lift on a count of two, lower on a count of four.)

Endurance: 2 sets of 12 to 15 reps.

Power: Tuesday: Power group A exercises (1 × 10, 1 × 8, 1 × 6), the rest as in Endurance.
Friday: Power group B exercises (1 × 10, 1 × 8, 1 × 6), the rest as in Endurance.

Chisel: 2 sets of 12 reps. (Lift and lower on a count of two.)

Marathon Basic

WEEK	MONDAY	TUESDAY	WEDNESDAY	THURSDAY	In Min.	FRIDAY	SATURDAY	In Min.	SATURDAY	SUNDAY	In Min.	TOTAL In Min.
	Run Easy Recovery in Min.	Warm-up/ Weights	Run Moderate Aerobic/Endurance in Min.	Run High Aerobic or Speed		Rest/ Run Endurance	Run Moderate Aerobic		Warm-up/ Weights	Run Endurance		
1 EASY	30	OFF	30		25	OFF		25	OFF		60	170
2	30	ADA 1×12	35		30	OFF		30	ADA 1×12		80	205
3	30	ADA 1×12	40		35	OFF		25	ADA 1×15		90	220
4 RECOVERY	30	ADA 1×15	35		30	OFF	10×10SEC. SURGES	20	OFF	10K RACE	50	165
5	30	END 2×12	40		35	OFF		35	END 2×12		100	240
6	30	END 2×12	45		40	OFF		40	END 2×12		110	265
7 RECOVERY	40	END 2×15	40		35	OFF		25	END 2×15		100	240
8	40	END 2×15	50		45	OFF		45	END 2×15		120	300
9	40	END 2×15	55		50	OFF	10×10SEC. SURGES	20	OFF	1/2 MARATHON	120	285
10 BEGIN SPEED	40	END 2×15	50	8×400	45	OFF		25	END 2×15		100	260
11	40	POW A	60	1×1MI., 1×800, 2×400, 3×100	50	OFF		40	POW B		130	320
12	40	POW A	40	3×5MIN. HILLS	50	OFF		45	POW B		150	325
13 RECOVERY	40	POW A	40	8×400, 8×100	50	OFF		25	POW B		110	265
14 LONGEST WEEK	40	CHI 2×12	30	3×3MIN., 1×9MIN., 3×2MIN. HILLS	50	OFF		45	CHI 2×12		170	335
15 BEGIN TAPER	30	CHI 2×12	40	3×1000, 3×400, 4×100	50	OFF		50	CHI 2×12		100	270
16	30	OFF	40	5×90SEC., 5×30SEC. HILLS	40	OFF	10×10SEC. SURGES	20	OFF	10K RACE	50	180
17	30	OFF	OFF	2×1MI. STRAIGHTS & CURVES	40	OFF		25	OFF		75	170
18	25	OFF	30	EASY	20	OFF	10×10SEC. SURGES	20	OFF	MARATHON	240	335

Key

ADA=Adaptation, **END**=Endurance, **POW**=Power, **CHI**=Chisel

Easy Recovery: These are for recovery at heart rates at the very low end of aerobic ranges, approximately 20 to 30 beats below your Maximum Aerobic Heart Rate (MAHR).

Moderate Aerobic: Runs keeping your heart rate from 20 to 30 beats below up to a heart rate of 5 beats below your MAHR.

High Aerobic: The bulk of the workout, once warmed up, is held within 10 beats of your MAHR.

Endurance: Heart rates from 20 to 30 below your MAHR up to it.

Speed: Heart rates above your MAHR. Warm up for 10 to 15 minutes, gradually increasing speed and heart rate. Then, for each interval, continue to increase your heart rate, trying to get it above your MAHR on the first one and increasing it a beat or two for each one after that. The rest between should be enough to let your heart rate drop at least as low as your MAHR, if not 20 to 30 below it. *Straights and curves:* Run the straight sections of a running track fast, then jog more slowly around the curves.

WEEK	MONDAY	TUESDAY	WEDNESDAY	THURSDAY	In Min.	FRIDAY	SATURDAY	In Min.	SATURDAY	SUNDAY	In Min.	TOTAL In Min.
	Run Easy Recovery in Min.	Warm-up/ Weights	Run Moderate Aerobic/ Endurance in Min.	Run High Aerobic or Speed		Rest/Run Endurance	Run Moderate Aerobic		Warm-up/ Weights	Run Endurance		
1	30	OFF	40		40	OFF		30	OFF		80	220
2	30	ADA 1×12	45		30	OFF		30	ADA 1×12		90	225
3	30	ADA 1×12	50		35	60		25	ADA 1×15		100	300
4 RECOVERY	30	ADA 1×15	75		30	OFF	10×10SEC. SURGES	30	OFF	10K RACE	40	205
5	30	END 2×12	40		35	60		35	END 2×12		110	310
6	30	END 2×12	45		40	70		40	END 2×12		120	345
7 RECOVERY	40	END 2×15	40		35	OFF		25	END 2×15		110	250
8	40	END 2×15	50		45	80		40	END 2×15		135	310
9	40	END 2×15	55		50	OFF	10×10SEC. SURGES	20	OFF	1/2 MARATHON	90	255
10 BEGIN SPEED	40	END 2×15	60	8×400, 8×100	45	OFF		25	END 2×15		120	290
11	40	POW A	70	1×1MI., 2×800, 4×400, 6×100	50	OFF		40	POW B		150	350
12	40	POW A	50	4×5MIN. HILLS	80	OFF		45	POW B		170	385
13 RECOVERY	40	POW A	60	8×400, 8×100	50	OFF		25	POW B		120	295
14 LONGEST RUN	40	CHI 2×12	30	3×4MIN., 1×9MIN., 3×3MIN. HILLS	90	OFF		45	CHI 2×12		180	385
15 BEGIN TAPER	30	CHI 2×12	50	3×1000,4×400, 8×100	60	OFF		50	CHI 2×12		110	300
16	30	OFF	40	5×90SEC., 5×30SEC. HILLS	45	OFF	10×10SEC. SURGES	30	OFF	10K RACE	40	185
17	30	OFF	40	2×1MI. STRAIGHTS & CURVES		OFF		25	OFF		75	170
18	30	OFF	40	EASY	25	OFF	10×10SEC. SURGES	20	OFF	MARATHON	180	295

Key

ADA=Adaptation, END=Endurance, POW=Power, CHI=Chisel

Easy Recovery: These are for recovery at heart rates at the very low end of aerobic ranges, approximately 20 to 30 beats below your Maximum Aerobic Heart Rate (MAHR).

Moderate Aerobic: Runs with your heart rate from 20 to 30 beats below up to a heart rate of 5 beats below your MAHR.

High Aerobic: The bulk of the workout, once warmed up, is held within 10 beats of your MAHR.

Endurance: Heart rates from 20 to 30 below your MAHR up to it.

Speed: Heart rates above your MAHR. Warm up for 10 to 15 minutes, gradually increasing speed and heart rate. Then, for each interval, continue to increase your heart rate, trying to get it above your MAHR on the first one and increasing it a beat or two for each one after that. The rest between should be enough to let your heart rate drop at least as low as your MAHR, if not 20 to 30 below it. *Straights and curves:* Run the straight sections of a running track fast, then jog more slowly around the curves.

WEEK TO RACE	WEEK	MONDAY	TUESDAY	WEDNESDAY	THURSDAY	FRIDAY	SATURDAY	SUNDAY
18	1	OFF	OFF	OFF	OFF	OFF	OFF	
17	2	OFF	ADA	OFF	OFF	ADA	OFF	
16	3	OFF	ADA	OFF	OFF	ADA	OFF	
15	4 RECOVERY	OFF	ADA	OFF	OFF	OFF	OFF	10K RACE
14	5	OFF	END	OFF	OFF	END	OFF	
13	6	OFF	END	OFF	OFF	END	OFF	
12	7 RECOVERY	OFF	END	OFF	OFF	END	OFF	
11	8	OFF	END	OFF	OFF	END	OFF	
10	9	OFF	END	OFF	OFF	OFF	OFF	1/2 MARATHON
9	10 BEGIN SPEED	OFF	END	OFF	OFF	END	OFF	
8	11	OFF	POW	OFF	OFF	POW	OFF	
7	12	OFF	POW	OFF	OFF	POW	OFF	
6	13 RECOVERY	OFF	POW	OFF	OFF	POW	OFF	
5	14 LONGEST RUN	OFF	CHI	OFF	OFF	CHI	OFF	
4	15 BEGIN TAPER	OFF	CHI	OFF	OFF	CHI	OFF	
3	16	OFF	OFF	OFF	OFF	OFF	OFF	10K RACE
2	17	OFF	OFF	OFF	OFF	OFF	OFF	
1	18	OFF	OFF	OFF	OFF	OFF	OFF	MARATHON

Key

ADA=Adaptation, **END**=Endurance, **POW**=Power, **CHI**=Chisel

Adaptation: 1 set of 12 to 15 reps. (Lift on a count of two, lower on a count of four.)

Endurance: 2 sets of 12 to 15 reps.

Power: Tuesday: Power group A exercises (1 × 10, 1 × 8, 1 × 6), the rest as in Endurance
Friday: Power group B exercises (1 × 10, 1 × 8, 1 × 6), the rest as in Endurance

Chisel: 2 sets of 12 reps. (Lift and lower on a count of two.)

Ironman Basic

WEEK	MONDAY Moderate Aerobic in Yards	TUESDAY Rest	WEDNESDAY Endurance in Yards	THURSDAY Rest	FRIDAY High Aerobic or Speed	SATURDAY Off or Easy	In Yards	SUNDAY Rest or Race	In Yards	TOTAL In Yards
SWIM										
1 EASY	2000	OFF	2500	OFF	2500	OFF		OFF		7000
2	2500	OFF	3000	OFF	2500	OFF		OFF		8000
3	2500	OFF	3500	OFF	3000	OFF		OFF		9000
4 RECOVERY	2500	OFF	3000	OFF	OFF	10×10SEC. SURGES	500	OLYMPIC DISTANCE	1500	7500
5	1000	OFF	3500	OFF	3000	OFF		OFF		7500
6	3000	OFF	4000	OFF	3000	OFF		OFF		10000
7 RECOVERY	3000	OFF	3000	OFF	2500	OFF		OFF		8500
8	3500	OFF	4500	OFF	2500	OFF		OFF		10500
9	2500	OFF	3000	OFF	OFF	10×10SEC. SURGES	500	1/2 IRONMAN	2000	8000
10 BEGIN SPEED	1000	OFF	3500	OFF	2500	OFF		OFF		7000
11	3000	OFF	4000	OFF	3000	OFF		OFF		10000
12	3500	OFF	5000	OFF	3000	OFF		OFF		11500
13 RECOVERY	3000	OFF	3500	OFF	2500	OFF		OFF		9000
14 LONGEST WEEK	4000	OFF	5500	OFF	3000	OFF		OFF		12500
15 BEGIN TAPER	3000	OFF	3500	OFF	2500	OFF		OFF		9000
16	2500	OFF	3000	OFF	OFF	10×10SEC. SURGES	500	OLYMPIC DISTANCE	1500	7500
17	2000	OFF	3000	OFF	3500	OFF		OFF		8500
18	1500	OFF	2000	OFF	OFF	10×10SEC. SURGES	500	IRONMAN	4000	8000

Key

Easy Recovery: These are for recovery at heart rates at the very low end of aerobic ranges, approximately 20 to 30 beats below your Maximum Aerobic Heart Rate (MAHR).

Moderate Aerobic: Swims keeping your heart rate from 20 to 30 beats below up to a heart rate of 5 beats below your MAHR.

High Aerobic: For the bulk of the workout, once warmed up, you keep your heart rate within 10 beats of your MAHR.

Endurance: Heart rates from 20 to 30 below your MAHR up to it.

Speed: Heart rates above your MAHR. Warm up for 10 to 15 minutes, gradually increasing speed and heart rate. Then, for each interval, continue to increase your heart rate, trying to get it above your MAHR on the first one and increasing it a beat or two for each one after that. The rest between should be enough to let your heart rate drop at least as low as your MAHR if not 20 to 30 below it.

WEEK	MONDAY	TUESDAY Moderate Aerobic Endurance in Min.	WEDNESDAY	THURSDAY High Aerobic or Speed	In Min.	FRIDAY	SATURDAY Endurance	In Min.	SUNDAY Rest or Race	In Min.	TOTAL In Min.
BIKE	Rest		Rest			Rest					
1 EASY	OFF	60	OFF		60	OFF		120		OFF	240
2	OFF	60	OFF		90	OFF		150		OFF	300
3	OFF	60	OFF		90	OFF		180		OFF	330
4 RECOVERY	OFF	60	OFF		60	OFF	10×10SEC. SURGES	30	OLYMPIC DISTANCE	90	240
5	OFF	60	OFF		90	OFF		180		OFF	330
6	OFF	60	OFF		90	OFF		210		OFF	360
7 RECOVERY	OFF	60	OFF		60	OFF		180		OFF	300
8	OFF	120	OFF		90	OFF		240		OFF	450
9	OFF	120	OFF		60	OFF	10×10SEC. SURGES	30	1/2 IRONMAN	210	420
10 BEGIN SPEED	OFF	60	OFF	10×1 MIN.	60	OFF		210		OFF	330
11	OFF	90	OFF	1×5MIN., 5×2MIN.	60	OFF		270		OFF	420
12	OFF	120	OFF	3×5MIN. HILLS	90	OFF		300		OFF	510
13 RECOVERY	OFF	60	OFF	10×2MIN.	60	OFF		240		OFF	360
14 LONGEST WEEK	OFF	150	OFF	1×20MIN. HILLS OR TIME TRIAL	75	OFF		330		OFF	555
15 BEGIN TAPER	OFF	120	OFF	3×3MIN., 2×2MIN, 4×1MIN.	90	OFF		300		OFF	510
16	OFF	120	OFF	5×90SEC., 5×30SEC. HILLS	60	OFF	10×10SEC. SURGES	30	OLYMPIC DISTANCE	90	300
17	OFF	90	OFF	1×5MIN., 4×1MIN.	60	OFF		180		OFF	330
18	OFF	60	OFF	EASY	45	OFF	10×10SEC. SURGES	30	IRONMAN	420	555

Key

Easy Recovery: These are for recovery at heart rates at the very low end of aerobic ranges, approximately 20 to 30 beats below your Maximum Aerobic Heart Rate (MAHR).

Moderate Aerobic: Bike rides keeping your heart rate from 20 to 30 beats below up to a heart rate of 5 beats below your MAHR.

High Aerobic: For the bulk of the workout, once warmed up, you keep your heart rate within 10 beats of your MAHR.

Endurance: Heart rates from 20 to 30 below your MAHR up to it.

Speed: Heart rates above your MAHR. Warm up for 10 to 15 minutes, gradually increasing speed and heart rate. Then, for each interval, continue to increase your heart rate, trying to get it above your MAHR on the first one and increasing it a beat or two for each one after that. The rest between should be enough to let your heart rate drop at least as low as your MAHR if not 20 to 30 below it.

Ironman Basic

WEEK	MONDAY	TUESDAY	WEDNESDAY	THURSDAY	FRIDAY	In Min.	SATURDAY	In Min.	SUNDAY	In Min.	TOTAL In Min.
RUN	Easy Recovery in Min.	Rest	Moderate Aerobic/Endurance in Min.	Rest	High Aerobic or Speed		Rest or Race Prep		Endurance		
1 EASY	30	OFF	30	OFF		25	OFF			60	145
2	30	OFF	35	OFF		30	OFF			80	175
3	30	OFF	40	OFF	OFF			35		75	180
4 RECOVERY	30	OFF	35	OFF	OFF		10×10SEC. SURGES	20	OLYMPIC DISTANCE	50	135
5	30	OFF	40	OFF		35	OFF			100	205
6	30	OFF	45	OFF	OFF			40		110	225
7 RECOVERY	40	OFF	40	OFF		35	OFF			100	215
8	40	OFF	50	OFF	OFF			30		70	190
9	40	OFF	30	OFF	OFF		10×10SEC. SURGES	20	1/2 IRONMAN	120	215
10 BEGIN SPEED	30	OFF	30	OFF	8×400	45	OFF			80	185
11	40	OFF	55	OFF	1×1MI., 1×800, 2×400, 3×100	50	OFF			130	275
12	40	OFF	60	OFF	3×5MIN. HILLS	50	OFF			150	290
13 RECOVERY	30	OFF	40	OFF	8×400, 8×100	50	OFF			110	220
14 LONGEST WEEK	35	OFF	70	OFF	3×3MIN., 1×9MIN., 3×2MIN. HILLS	50		30		180	355
15 BEGIN TAPER	30	OFF	45	OFF	2×1000, 3×400, 4×100	50	OFF			100	215
16	OFF	OFF	25	OFF	5×90SEC., 5×30SEC. HILLS	OFF	10×10SEC. SURGES	20	OLYMPIC DISTANCE	50	175
17	30	OFF	30	OFF	2×1MI. STRAIGHTS & CURVES	40		60	OFF		160
18	25	OFF	30	OFF	OFF		10×10SEC. SURGES	20	IRONMAN	240	315

Key

Easy Recovery: These are for recovery at heart rates at the very low end of aerobic ranges, approximately 20 to 30 beats below your Maximum Aerobic Heart Rate (MAHR).

Moderate Aerobic: Runs keeping your heart rate from 20 to 30 beats below up to a heart rate of 5 beats below your MAHR.

High Aerobic: The bulk of the workout, once warmed up, is held within 10 beats of your MAHR.

Endurance: Heart rates from 20 to 30 below your MAHR up to it.

Speed: Heart rates above your MAHR. Warm up for 10 to 15 minutes, gradually increasing speed and heart rate. Then, for each interval, continue to increase your heart rate, trying to get it above your MAHR on the first one and increasing it a beat or two for each one after that. The rest between should be enough to let your heart rate drop at least as low as your MAHR, if not 20 to 30 below it.

Ironman Advanced

WEEK SWIM	MONDAY Moderate Aerobic in Yards	TUESDAY Rest	WEDNESDAY Endurance in Yards	THURSDAY Rest	FRIDAY High Aerobic or Speed in Yards	SATURDAY Off or Easy	In Yards	SUNDAY Rest or Race	In Yards	TOTAL In Yards
1 EASY	2500	OFF	3000	OFF	2500	OFF		OFF		8000
2	2500	OFF	3500	OFF	3000	OFF		OFF		9000
3	3000	OFF	4000	OFF	3000	OFF		EASY	1500	11500
4 RECOVERY	2500	OFF	3000	OFF	OFF	10×10SEC. SURGES	500	OLYMPIC DISTANCE	1500	7500
5	1500	OFF	4000	OFF	3000	OFF		OFF		8500
6	3000	OFF	4500	OFF	3500	OFF		EASY	2000	13000
7 RECOVERY	3000	OFF	3500	OFF	3000	OFF		OFF		9500
8	3500	OFF	5000	OFF	3000	OFF		EASY	1500	13000
9	2500	OFF	3000	OFF	OFF	10×10SEC. SURGES	500	1/2 IRONMAN	2000	8000
10 BEGIN SPEED	1500	OFF	3500	OFF	2500	OFF		OFF		7500
11	3000	OFF	4500	OFF	3000	OFF		OFF		10500
12	3500	OFF	5500	OFF	3500	OFF		EASY	2000	14500
13 RECOVERY	3000	OFF	4000	OFF	3000	OFF		OFF		10000
14 LONGEST WEEK	4500	OFF	6000	OFF	3000	OFF		EASY	2500	16000
15 BEGIN TAPER	3000	OFF	4000	OFF	3000	OFF			1500	11500
16	3000	OFF	3500	OFF	OFF	10×10SEC. SURGES	500	OLYMPIC DISTANCE	1500	8500
17	2000	OFF	3000	OFF	4000	OFF		OFF		9000
18	1500	OFF	2000	OFF	OFF	10×10SEC. SURGES	500	IRONMAN	4000	8000

Key

Easy Recovery: These are for recovery at heart rates at the very low end of aerobic ranges, approximately 20 to 30 beats below your Maximum Aerobic Heart Rate (MAHR).

Moderate Aerobic: Swims keeping your heart rate from 20 to 30 beats below up to a heart rate of 5 beats below your MAHR.

High Aerobic: For the bulk of the workout, once warmed up, you keep your heart rate within 10 beats of your MAHR.

Endurance: Heart rates from 20 to 30 below your MAHR up to it.

Speed: Heart rates above your MAHR. Warm up for 10 to 15 minutes, gradually increasing speed and heart rate. Then, for each interval, continue to increase your heart rate, trying to get it above your MAHR on the first one and increasing it a beat or two for each one after that. The rest between should be enough to let your heart rate drop at least as low as your MAHR, if not 20 to 30 below it.

Ironman Advanced

WEEK	MONDAY	TUESDAY	WEDNESDAY	THURSDAY	In Min.	FRIDAY	SATURDAY	In Min.	SUNDAY	In Min.	TOTAL
BIKE	Rest/Easy	Moderate Aerobic/ Endurance in Min.	Rest	High Aerobic or Speed	In Min.	Rest	Endurance	In Min.	Rest or Race	In Min.	In Min.
1 EASY	OFF	60	OFF		60	OFF		150	OFF		270
2	OFF	60	OFF		90	OFF		180	OFF		330
3	OFF	90	OFF		150	OFF		210	EASY	60	510
4 RECOVERY	OFF	120	OFF		60	OFF	10×10SEC. SURGES	30	OLYMPIC DISTANCE	75	285
5	OFF	60	OFF		120	OFF		240	OFF		420
6	OFF	60	OFF		210	OFF		270	EASY	60	600
7 RECOVERY	OFF	60	OFF		90	OFF		210	OFF		360
8	OFF	150	OFF		90	OFF		240	EASY	60	540
9	OFF	90	OFF		60	OFF	10×10SEC. SURGES	30	1/2 IRONMAN	180	360
10 BEGIN SPEED	OFF	60	OFF	10×1MIN.	60	OFF		210	OFF		330
11	OFF	120	OFF	1×5MIN., 5×2MIN.	60	OFF		300	OFF		480
12	OFF	150	OFF	3×5MIN. HILLS	90	OFF		360	EASY	60	660
13 RECOVERY	OFF	75	OFF	10×2MIN.	60	OFF		270	OFF		405
14 LONGEST WEEK	OFF	150	OFF	1×20MIN. HILLS OR TIME TRIAL	75	OFF		390	EASY	60	675
15 BEGIN TAPER	OFF	120	OFF	3×3MIN., 2×2MIN., 4×1MIN.	90	OFF		300	OFF		510
16	OFF	120	OFF	5×90SEC., 5×30SEC. HILLS	60	OFF	10×10SEC. SURGES	30	OLYMPIC DISTANCE	75	285
17	OFF	90	OFF	1×5MIN., 4×2MIN.	60	OFF		210	EASY	45	405
18	OFF	60	OFF	EASY	45	OFF	10×10SEC. SURGES	30	IRONMAN	360	495

Key

Easy Recovery: These are for recovery at heart rates at the very low end of aerobic ranges, approximately 20 to 30 beats below your Maximum Aerobic Heart Rate (MAHR).

Moderate Aerobic: Bike rides keeping your heart rate from 20 to 30 beats below up to a heart rate of 5 beats below your MAHR.

High Aerobic: For the bulk of the workout, once warmed up, you keep your heart rate within 10 beats of your MAHR.

Endurance: Heart rates from 20 to 30 below your MAHR up to it.

Speed: Heart rates above your MAHR. Warm up for 10 to 15 minutes, gradually increasing speed and heart rate. Then, for each interval, continue to increase your heart rate, trying to get it above your MAHR on the first one and increasing it a beat or two for each one after that. The rest between should be enough to let your heart rate drop at least as low as your MAHR if not 20 to 30 below it.

Ironman Advanced

WEEK	MONDAY	TUESDAY	WEDNESDAY	THURSDAY	FRIDAY	In Min.	SATURDAY	In Min.	SUNDAY	In Min.	TOTAL
RUN	Easy Recovery in Min.	Rest	Moderate Aerobic/Endurance in Min.	High Aerobic or Speed	High Aerobic or Speed	In Min.	Rest or Race Prep	In Min.	Endurance Min.		In Min.
1 EASY	30	OFF	40	OFF		25	OFF			75	170
2	30	OFF	50	OFF		30	OFF			90	200
3	30	OFF	45	OFF	OFF			35		80	190
4 RECOVERY	30	OFF	40	OFF	OFF		10×10SEC. SURGES	20	OLYMPIC DISTANCE	40	130
5	30	OFF	40	OFF		35	OFF			100	205
6	40	OFF	55	OFF	OFF		AFTER BIKE 40			120	255
7 RECOVERY	30	OFF	45	OFF		40	AFTER BIKE 45			110	230
8	40	OFF	45	OFF		35	OFF			90	210
9	40	OFF	35	OFF	OFF		10×10SEC. SURGES	20	1/2 IRONMAN	90	185
10 BEGIN SPEED	30	OFF	40	OFF	8×400, 8×100	45	OFF			90	205
11	40	OFF	60	OFF	1×1 MI., 2×800, 4×400, 6×100	50	OFF			135	285
12	40	OFF	75	OFF	4×5MIN. HILLS	50	AFTER BIKE 40			165	370
13 RECOVERY	40	OFF	45	OFF	8×400, 8×100	50	OFF			110	245
14 LONGEST WEEK	40	OFF	100	OFF	3×4MIN., 1×9MIN., 3×3MIN. HILLS	60	AFTER BIKE 45			180	425
15 BEGIN TAPER	30	OFF	45	OFF	3×1000, 4×400, 8×100	50	OFF			100	225
16	OFF	OFF	90	OFF	5×90SEC., 5×30SEC. HILLS	OFF	10×10SEC. SURGES	20	OLYMPIC DISTANCE	40	180
17	30	90	25	OFF	2×1MI. STRAIGHTS & CURVES	40		75	OFF		220
18	30	OFF	35	OFF	OFF		10×10SEC. SURGES	20	IRONMAN	210	295

Key

Easy Recovery: These are for recovery at heart rates at the very low end of aerobic ranges, approximately 20 to 30 beats below your Maximum Aerobic Heart Rate (MAHR).

Moderate Aerobic: Runs with your heart rate from 20 to 30 beats below up to a heart rate of 5 beats below your MAHR.

High Aerobic: The bulk of the workout, once warmed up, is held within 10 beats of your MAHR.

Endurance: Heart rates from 20 to 30 below your MAHR up to it.

Speed: Heart rates above your MAHR. Warm up for 10 to 15 minutes, gradually increasing speed and heart rate. Then, for each interval, continue to increase your heart rate, trying to get it above your MAHR on the first one and increasing it a beat or two for each one after that. The rest between should be enough to let your heart rate drop at least as low as your MAHR if not 20 to 30 below it.

Ironman Weights

WEEK TO RACE	WEEK	MONDAY	TUESDAY	WEDNESDAY	THURSDAY	FRIDAY	SATURDAY	SUNDAY
18	1	OFF	OFF	OFF	OFF	OFF	OFF	
17	2	OFF	ADA 1×12	OFF	OFF	ADA 1×12	OFF	
16	3	OFF	ADA 1×12	OFF	OFF	ADA 1×15	OFF	
15	4 RECOVERY	OFF	ADA 1×15	OFF	OFF	OFF	OFF	OLYMPIC DISTANCE
14	5	OFF	END 2×12	OFF	OFF	END 2×12	OFF	
13	6	OFF	END 2×12	OFF	OFF	END 2×12	OFF	
12	7 RECOVERY	OFF	END 2×15	OFF	OFF	END 2×15	OFF	
11	8	OFF	END 2×15	OFF	OFF	END 2×15	OFF	
10	9	OFF	END 2×15	OFF	OFF	OFF	OFF	1/2 IRONMAN
9	10 BEGIN SPEED	OFF	END 2×15	OFF	OFF	END 2×15	OFF	
8	11	OFF	POW A	OFF	OFF	POW B	OFF	
7	12	OFF	POW A	OFF	OFF	POW B	OFF	
6	13 RECOVERY	OFF	POW A	OFF	OFF	POW B	OFF	
5	14 LONGEST RUN	OFF	CHI 2×12	OFF	OFF	CHI 2×12	OFF	
4	15 BEGIN TAPER	OFF	CHI 2×12	OFF	OFF	CHI 2×12	OFF	
3	16	OFF	OFF	OFF	OFF	OFF	OFF	OLYMPIC DISTANCE
2	17	OFF	OFF	OFF	OFF	OFF	OFF	
1	18	OFF	OFF	OFF	OFF	OFF	OFF	IRONMAN

Key

ADA=Adaptation, **END**=Endurance, **POW**=Power, **CHI**=Chisel

Adaptation: 1 set of 12 to 15 reps. (Lift on a count of two, lower on a count of four.)

Endurance: 2 sets of 12 to 15 reps.

Power: Tuesday: Power group A exercises (1 × 10, 1 × 8, 1 × 6), the rest as in Endurance .
Friday: Power group B exercises (1 × 10, 1 × 8, 1 × 6), the rest as in Endurance.

Chisel: 2 sets of 12 reps. (Lift and lower on a count of two.)

Part III

Get
Healthy

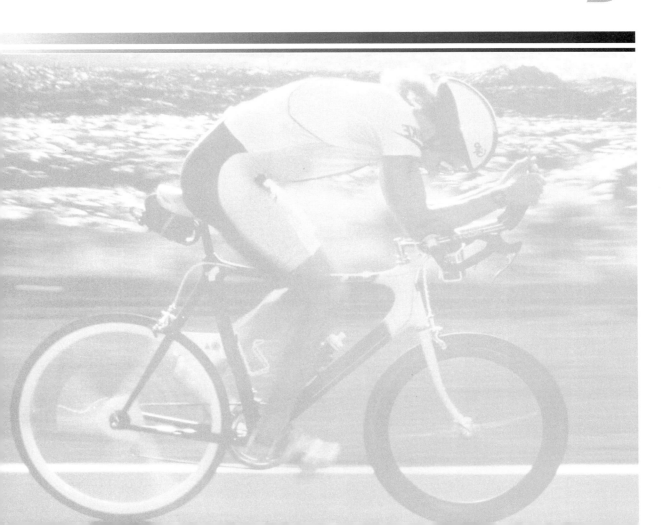

9 Nutrition—How to Make Food Really Work for You

Let's start with the brain. This organ, above all others in your body, calls the shots. It's pretty obvious that without a brain you would not function, even though you probably know someone who seems to function without one anyway. The brain has one—and only one—fuel it can use to keep it purring along smoothly. That magic substance is a simple sugar called *glucose.*

Glucose doesn't just appear in your brain. It is served up at the brain's dining table through the nonstop steady pipeline called the bloodstream. This cerebral room service is very precise. The brain is somewhat of a prima donna—it is happy only if it gets its glucose at a very specific rate. If it gets too much too fast, the brain revolts and starts to go haywire. If the service is too slow,

and the brain doesn't get enough glucose quickly enough, it panics. The brain does not like either of these states and starts screaming at the rest of the body to fix it whenever these situations happen.

- When you eat carbohydrates, a substance called *serotonin* is released. Serotonin calms the brain down, which is great for sleeping but not very good for thinking.

- The opposite happens when you eat protein. This causes *norepinephrine* to be released, which stimulates the brain. This is a good thing if you need clear, alert thinking.

The rest of the body doesn't really like it when the brain gets angry. To keep the brain from yelling, the bloodstream has a few helpers who do their best to keep the delivery service exactly on schedule with glucose to the boss upstairs. The two main helpers that regulate the amount of glucose in the bloodstream are *insulin* and *glucagon*.

Insulin is a hormone your pancreas produces when the brain is getting too much glucose too quickly. It drags glucose out of the bloodstream, which in effect slows down the service of the sugar to the brain. But insulin has to do something with the excess sugar it's pulling out of the bloodstream. It has two choices.

The first option is to convert the glucose into another form of carbohydrate called *glycogen*. This is deposited in your liver and muscles for use later as fuel for the brain or for muscular activity when you exercise. You can store about 2,000 calories' worth of glycogen through this process. After that, the deposit slots for glycogen are full. Insulin then goes to option two, which is to take the excess blood glucose, convert it to fat, and deposit it in the most unsightly places, like saddlebags and other fat colonies throughout the body.

Once the empty containers for glycogen are filled, it doesn't matter how low in fat your diet is. Any further intake of carbohydrates will be stored as fat. Period.

While insulin helps the brain out when glucose is arriving too quickly, glucagon remedies the opposite problem. When not enough glucose is arriving to keep the brain happy, glucagon goes to where glycogen is stored, pulls some out, converts it back into glucose, then spits it back out into the bloodstream, where it is transported up to the hungry brain for fuel. In addition to mobilizing glycogen, glucagon is responsible for grabbing fat from storage and making it available to the body as fuel. Glucagon also opens up your blood vessels, which makes it easier to deliver oxygen to all the cells in your body.

You have enough energy stored as glycogen to run about 20 miles. The amount of fat in your body could propel you from San Diego to San Francisco, a distance of about 500 miles!

There's Always a Downside Insulin and glucagon are partners working in opposite ways to keep the brain happy. It sounds foolproof, but there are some potentially bad side effects to the equation.

Eating excess amounts of complex carbohydrates like breads and pastas, or eating even moderate amounts of simple sugars like those used to sweeten Grandma's berry pie, cause blood sugar levels to skyrocket. This causes huge amounts of insulin to be released, which stops fat burning.

If the brain is overloaded with glucose coming at it from the bloodstream, a situation caused by eating too many carbohydrates or by overeating in general, insulin release is switched to overdrive. This turns off the production of glucagon, causing a metabolic traffic jam. If insulin is high, glucagon production is shut down, blood vessels constrict, slowing the delivery of oxygen to cells, and fat burning is blocked.

It takes more oxygen to break down fat than carbohydrate for use as energy. Therefore, anything that causes vasoconstriction (one of the side effects of insulin release) slows down the delivery of oxygen to the cells for metabolic processes and ultimately inhibits fat metabolism.

The second negative reaction in this chain of events is that high insulin levels usually do their job too well, which means that the system overcompensates in storing glucose, causing blood glucose levels to fall below the preference of your brain. Since glucagon production is also blocked, the only way to raise blood glucose levels back up is to munch on something sweet.

If insulin stores more sugar than necessary, the brain is starved for glucose. It can't get enough from the blood, and glucagon won't help to release some because the excess insulin floating around turns off its production. The brain is freaking out. To the outside world, a person in this state will look either sleepy and lethargic (not enough glucose to fire the brain properly), or like a raving maniac panicking because the brain wants the person to eat something sweet and bring the glucose levels back up right away. Either way, this is not a balanced state for your body to be in.

Stay in the Zone Once the fat burning is shut off, it doesn't come back to full power for *seven to nine hours.* You may have had a great aerobic workout earlier in the day, but if you follow it with a big dose of simple carbohydrates, physiologically you look like you did an anaerobic session—fat burning is shut down.

The following is a summary of how insulin and glucagon work in your body:

EFFECT ON	INSULIN	GLUCAGON
Blood glucose	Lowers	Raises
Blood vessels	Vasoconstricts	Vasodilates
Fat metabolism	Turns off fat burning	Turns on fat burning
Human growth hormone	Depresses release	
Cholesterol	Raises levels	
Immune system	Depresses	

In the long run, it's better to keep blood sugar in the correct zone for the brain, instead of relying on hormones to go into action to correct an extreme situation. There are two ways to do this. One is through eating the right balance of foods. The other is by exercising.

Balancing Your Diet Just about everything you ingest will affect this balance. Excess caffeine, for example, can stimulate an overproduction of insulin and put a huge stress on your adrenal system. The goal is to eat and drink the foods that support the balance in your body, especially the ones that affect the blood sugar balance. Two types of foods do this through their influence on insulin and glucagon: carbohydrates and proteins. Eat a bunch of carbohydrates, and insulin levels will rise. Eat small to moderate amounts of protein, and glucagon will rise. Fats don't do either of these things directly. However, if fats are eaten with carbohydrates, they will slow the rate of absorption, reducing the insulin response from that carbohydrate.

Exercise has a similar impact on stabilizing blood sugar levels. Aerobic (cardiovascular) exercise does two things: It decreases insulin levels and it increases glucagon levels, both of which are desirable. The end result is that your body's rate of fat burning is increased, which is exactly what most people are trying to do through starvation diets and other methods of weight loss. In fact, 95 percent of all people who diet gain back the weight they lose, and more, within five years!

Here is another plus to working out. There is a metabolic response to exercise in the muscles for up to forty-eight hours after exercise. So even though you may only burn 500 calories during a 5-mile run, the *total* calories burned because of the workout will be more, due to a temporary increase in your metabolic rate.

Anaerobic exercise, such as weight lifting, stimulates the pituitary gland to release human growth hormone (HGH), the most powerful fat-burning hormone in your body. In addition to kicking fat burning into high gear, HGH is required for building new muscle fiber and repairing damaged muscle after a workout.

HGH does its job at night while you sleep. No sleep, no recovery. Another killer for HGH is insulin, which is another reason to avoid overeating carbohydrates. High insulin levels will keep your body from releasing HGH. No HGH, no recovery, and no new muscle can be laid down.

Mark: Sharing Meals Working together as a couple provides many of the positives that come from eating a balanced diet and getting enough sleep. It helps to have a partner—she's my good food conscience. We don't always work out at the same times, but we always have meals together. It is a joint effort all the way. I am probably stricter about following a healthy eating regime than Julie would be on her own. She can take just about any meal—no matter how dull—and modify it to be gourmet. So, together, we get the best of all worlds: health and great taste.

What the Glycemic Index Means The amount of insulin response caused by different rates of absorption of different foods has been measured. It is gauged by something called the glycemic index. Glucose is at the high end of the index, with a rating of 100. This means that eating a lot of glucose would stimulate a large amount of insulin to be released. At the other end of the spectrum are peanuts, with a glycemic index rating of about 15. This can actually reduce insulin.

FOOD	GLYCEMIC INDEX
Very High (100 +)	
Rice cake	132
French bread	131
Honey	126
Cornflakes	121
Mashed potato	117
Baked russet potato	116
Puffed wheat	110
White bread	100
Wheat bread	100
High (80–100)	
Corn chips	99
Carrots	93
Raisins	93
Ice cream (fat-free)	90
Yogurt (fat-free frozen)	90
Banana	82
Brown rice	81
Moderate (50–80)	
Oatmeal cookie	78
Yams	73
Orange juice	71
Ice cream (full fat)	69
Pinto beans	64
Low (30–50)	
Apple	49
Oatmeal	49
Grapes	45
Milk	44
Pear	34
Very Low (less than 30)	
Grapefruit	26
Plums	25
Cherries	23
Most vegetables	23
Soybeans	20
All nuts	15

Are you always hungry? Here are some troubleshooting steps to help curb the urge to munch before lunch.

• **Eat four to six smaller meals.** This keeps the calories going in at a steady rate throughout the day instead of letting your body deplete itself of available calories from a meal that may have been eaten six to eight hours earlier.

• **Make sure you are getting enough water.** Often a hunger signal will actually be your body asking for plain water.

• **Cut down on carbohydrates, cut out refined sugars, and raise your protein intake.** This will help keep blood sugar levels even and cut down on the chance that your brain will panic for its food.

Julie: Satisfying Your Hunger If you know you are getting enough calories to sustain your body weight and still feel hungry, ask yourself if there are reasons you are eating other than physical ones. Unhappiness, stress, dissatisfaction with your life can all manifest themselves in a hunger that does not ever become satiated with food.

Come up with positive alternatives to eating as a way to "make up" for whatever doesn't feel right in your life. I like to get a massage. Exercise is very good for this. In the long run, changing your job and priorities to come in line with what is important to you in your life is probably the best thing you can do to curb your hunger.

If you have deeper feelings or hurt that seem to permeate your being and self-image, maybe it's time to seek counseling. No amount of food will solve any of these problems for you.

The Carbohydrate Story You need carbohydrates. It's that simple. Yet it's important to find ones that don't cause a big release of insulin. In the simplest of terms, if a carbohydrate can get from your mouth to your brain in a short time, it will cause insulin to be released. The stomach just takes what you shove into it, breaks it down, and then sends it on its way. If you take in a sugar that breaks down quickly into glucose, away it goes like lightning to the brain. You know what happens next. The brain goes into its fit and stomps on the pancreas, which responds by spitting out a bunch of insulin.

Simple carbohydrates are usually the ones that cause this unwanted response. They come from starchy foods that are refined, and include all simple sugars such as Coke, Frosted Flakes, white bread, and just about every dessert you can think of. These are generally short-chain molecules that require little work by the stomach to prepare them for the bloodstream.

If it takes longer for the stomach to break down the carbohydrates you eat, they will enter the bloodstream more slowly. *Complex carbohydrates* are the ones that take this extra time. They are long-chain molecules, which take more work and time to break down than simple ones. They are found in whole grain breads, some fruits, vegetables, and beans. By eating a moderate amount of complex carbohydrates, you can avoid an insulin response and keep your body in the fat-burning zone.

Another way to slow their rate of absorption is to eat carbohydrates with proteins and/or fats. Fiber also slows down the speed at which they enter your bloodstream, which is one of the pluses of eating whole foods. You need about 10 grams of fiber for every 1,000 calories, or about 15 to 25g per day. You can get this in a cup of cooked black beans or pinto beans or in three pieces of fresh fruit each day.

There is a third type of carbohydrate called *gray area carbohydrates.* Examples are white rice and white pasta, some fruits, and even potatoes. These will make some people release insulin but not others, depending on how sensitive you are to blood sugar fluctuation. Unfortunately, in this area, we are not all created equal.

If you become lethargic or feel bloated after a normal serving of a gray area carbohydrate, you are probably sensitive to them and should stick with purely complex forms. If you feel good after eating these forms of carbohydrates and your energy levels don't drop, you can probably get away with the pasta of choice.

Mark: Changing Habits When I was racing, I gobbled down chocolate-chip cookies almost every day. Even though eating them didn't seem to affect my performance, I knew they were probably not good for me. First of all, even though they were so delicious, they filled me up with calories that did nothing for me.

Cookies didn't make me stronger or healthier. Secondly, I knew they were making my blood sugar go through some moderate swings, because I wanted more cookies a few hours after the last ones.

So I decided to give them up. I didn't know for how long, but I knew it had to be until I didn't crave them anymore. Once I made this decision, it was amazing the number of places that seemed to jump out at me where I could buy chocolate-chip cookies. It seemed as if there was a cookie vendor on every corner. Traveling became a nightmare. Airports seemed to be the mecca of cookie sellers. Every little weird airport shop had some for sale.

Time passed slowly, very slowly. Eventually, I could walk by a Mrs. Fields without feeling as if I were leaving my only child behind. Now, I rarely notice those cookie sellers at all.

Fats Fat is the latest hero of the foodies. For years, it was taboo to include more than a blip of fat in your diet. Fortunately, science has prevailed and you are once again able to eat fat guilt-free.

> *Essential fat comprises 3 to 5 percent of a man's body weight and 11 to 13 percent of a woman's.*

Fats are involved with just about every process in your body. They are necessary for cell membrane integrity, hormone production, energy metabolism, and proper heart function. A diet too low in fat will kill you just as quickly as a diet too high in fat. As with everything else you eat, there is a proper balance that will enable your body to be at its peak level of health and performance.

Three types of fats have to be eaten in the right balance: omega-6, saturated, and omega-3. Omega-6 fats are unsaturated and monounsaturated fats that come from vegetable sources like safflower, canola, and olive oils. Omega-3 fats, which are also unsaturated, come from fish (especially cold-water fish such as salmon), beans, soy, and walnuts. These two forms of fat are anti-inflammatory, lower blood pressure, and increase circulation.

You want a snack that supplies you with some of these essential fats? Eat a nut. One ounce of walnuts has one quarter of the daily requirement of vitamin E and omega-3 fats that are normally found in fish. One ounce is about fourteen walnut halves, twenty-four to thirty almonds, or thirty-five peanuts.

Saturated fats come from foods of animal origin (other than fish) and are also found in dairy products. This form of fat causes inflammation, decreases circulation, and raises blood pressure.

Another form of fat exists out there in the modern world that has no positive function whatsoever in your body. These are partially hydrogenated or trans fats. Avoid this form of fat at all costs. Trans fats lower HDL and raise both LDL and triglyceride levels in your blood, which leads to heart disease. If even a small percentage of your fats comes from trans fats (as little as 5 percent of your total fat intake), it can be enough to muck up the system.

Trans fats are found in almost every type of processed food on the market. Their use is valuable to the food industry because they are very stable, don't break down on the grocery-store shelf, and work exceptionally well as a food preservative. The problem with them is that they don't break down in your body, either. They stick around for a long time in your system. For athletes, one of their side effects is to increase your perception of pain!

These are tricky fats to spot. Reading the labels on products is the only way to be sure you avoid eating partially hydrogenated fats. Don't be misled by the claims on the front of a product. "No cholesterol" does *not* equate to "no

> *LDL carries fats made in your liver to body tissues. While it takes aerobic activity to raise the amount of HDL in your blood, it only takes moderate amounts of physical activity to lower your total cholesterol and LDL.*

partially hydrogenated fats." "No saturated fat" does *not* equate to "no partially hydrogenated fats." "Low in fat" does *not* equate to "no partially hydrogenated fats." Read the labels and don't make assumptions.

Taking healthy polyunsaturated fat like canola oil and converting it to partially hydrogenated fat makes it solid at room temperature. It's magic—margarine! However, small amounts of trans fats are more harmful than larger amounts of saturated fats. A small increase in saturated fats results in a 17 percent increase in coronary artery disease. A similar increase in trans fats leads to a 93 percent increase.

TYPE OF FAT	EFFECT IN THE BODY
Omega-3, -6	Lowers LDL
Unsaturated and mono-unsaturated fats	Increase circulation, decrease inflammation
Saturated fats	Lower HDL, raise LDL, decrease circulation, increase blood pressure, increase inflammation
Excess saturated fats	Cause insulin resistance
Trans fats (partially hydrogenated oils)	Raise LDL, lower HDL, raise triglycerides, increase perception of pain
Aerobic exercise	Raises HDL, lowers insulin levels
Excess anaerobic exercise	Lowers HDL

Why Eat Fat? Eating healthy fats is far healthier than eating no fats. A study by the *Journal of the American Medical Association* showed that men on low-fat diets actually fared worse than those on moderate-fat diets, with the low-fat group's HDL (good cholesterol) dropping and the harmful triglyceride levels rising.

Why? Most replaced the fat with carbohydrates. This lowers total cholesterol, but also lowers HDL levels, increasing heart-disease risk more than diets that replace saturated or trans fats with unsaturated fats. Exchanging

> *In a thirty-year study of 1,822 middle-aged men, those who ate the most fish— a little more than an ounce a day on average—were 38 percent less likely to die from heart disease and 44 percent less likely to have a heart attack than men who ate no fish.*

fats for carbs can also lead to diabetes by increasing blood insulin levels.

The final tidbit on fats is to avoid fried foods. Frying requires fats to be heated, which tends to make them rancid. Rancid fats have a lot of free radicals, which are like little atomic bombs floating inside of your body, causing cellular damage. Any spot on the cell membrane damaged by free radicals is a magnet for fatty deposits to build up on, which is one of the reasons people who eat a lot of fried foods get heart disease.

Protein Protein's main function is to be the building blocks for muscle tissue. An adequate amount is needed to build up your muscles after workouts tear them down. An endurance athlete may need more daily protein than a body builder.

Along with muscle building, protein helps stabilize your blood sugar levels during exercise and during rest. So, in addition to moderating your intake of simple carbohydrates and exercising, getting enough protein will keep your energy levels stable for long periods of time.

High-quality proteins come from animal sources (meat, fish, eggs, yogurt), or by combining grains with legumes in the same meal. Good combinations would be tortillas and beans or rice and lentils, for instance. Soy is the only protein in the vegetable kingdom that is considered to be complete, which means it has all of the essential amino acids your body needs to build new muscle tissue.

The choice of where you get your quality proteins is up to you.

One of the pluses for a vegetarian diet is the ease of regulating the normally high intake of saturated fats in the United States. Also, most vitamins and minerals are found in fruits and vegetables. The downside to a vegetarian diet is that most people who make this choice eat way too many carbohydrates and not enough protein. People on a vegetarian diet eat as much as 80 percent of their calories from carbohydrates and as little as 10 percent from protein. If you are a vegetarian, think protein, protein, and more protein.

How to Change a Bad Habit into a Good One Identify a dietary habit you want to change. Pick one that will require you to stop eating something, like ice cream after dinner. Identify a suitable substitute, in this case a piece of fruit or even just a little more of the well-rounded foods from dinner, and have it available for the craving hour.

• Set a goal period during which you will not, under any circumstances, give in. It takes about six weeks to change a very ingrained habit. Realize now that there will be endless opportunities where your favorite thing will be shoved in your face to tempt you.

• The initial ten to fifteen days will be the most difficult. Your body will crave whatever it is you have given up, but slowly your chemistry will balance out. Foods that may not have been very satisfying before will step in and become ambrosia.

• If you must, at the end of your test period, make a looser pact with yourself about adding the food back in on occasion. Occasional eating of something decadent is not a habit. Daily or many times over a day is a habit.

Water A lot of people weigh themselves after a workout and see their weight has dropped from say, 178 to 169, and they think "Great! I lost nine pounds." But a sudden weight drop might signal dehydration. Studies have shown that most athletes drink, at best, about half of what their bodies need.

Let's look at the reality of this exciting drop in weight. For a long run of 12 miles, you might easily expend 1,200 calories. (Most formulas for a 150-pound person calculate that running a mile takes 100 calories.) This should clue you in that most of that drop in weight is from water loss. If you replace the water you sweated out during that run, the actual loss of fat will be about one third of a pound.

If you lose 5 percent of your body weight from fluid loss, your performance drops 20 percent. If you were a car, you wouldn't want to be cruising around with the radiator half full. Make sure you carry water with you.

If you are cycling, add some extra water bottles on your bike in extreme heat. You might carry another extra bottle in your jersey or use a CamelBak or similar system. When running, put a water bottle in a fanny pack. If you have the time, go out before a long run and stash water bottles along your route so they will be available every twenty to thirty minutes. Scout out the water fountains along the way. In short, plan ahead.

It is important to replenish your body with fluids and nutrients quickly after your workout is completed. The first half hour after you are done is when your body has the greatest ability to absorb depleted nutrients and fluids. Hitting that window with the proper foods will speed recovery and increase fitness at a much greater rate.

Give your body fluids and nutrients in this order:

1. fluids
2. carbohydrates
3. proteins

This order goes from quickest to slowest in terms of absorption rates. It gives your body the

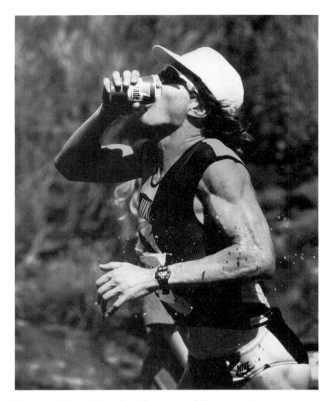

During a long day of racing or training, you become your own best temperature gauge. Mine is telling me that it is over one hundred degrees in the lava fields and I had better cool off and fuel up! Knowing the needs of your body is essential.

greatest chance of getting the full benefit out of each one.

Water Guidelines

• Drink eight 8-ounce glasses of water per day. Add an additional 4 ounces for every fifteen minutes of cardiovascular work you do.

• Drinking water before you work out helps lower your body's core temperature, reducing the added stress heat places on your cardiovascular system.

• How much water should you drink after exercise? Drink 1 pint for every pound you lost.

10 *Managing Your Diet*

The best guide for eating exactly the right amount of food is a forgotten adaptation you have built into your body. It's called an *appetite*. Eat when you are hungry and stop when you are full. It's simple enough to be guided by your appetite while eating all the calories and nutrients you need, in the absence of social eating pressures and the personal/emotional reasons you eat other than hunger.

If you don't believe your body is telling you what and how much to eat to achieve your goals, a few handy tips can guide you in the right direction.

Julie: Body Composition In 1998, I was training for the Rock 'n' Roll marathon here in San Diego. I wanted to add some muscle in ad-

dition to the running I was doing in hopes of having something extra to draw on in the race. So I went into the gym twice a week to work out with a strength coach.

After about twelve weeks, my muscle mass was going up, but there was absolutely no change in that winter layer of fat. Even with nearly 70 miles a week of running and all the weight work, I was not leaning out.

I started to get desperate and slipped back into my old college-days mentality of trying to lose weight by eating as little food as possible. A cup of coffee and two pieces of toast in the morning would be about it until dinnertime. Dinner always ended up as a pig-out session. I was overeating late in the day, plus I felt like I deserved a dessert (a *big* dessert) because I had worked out all day.

Breaking Even

The first task is to determine the amount of food that will sustain your body weight as it is right now. You can adjust that number up or down to reflect what you are trying to accomplish.

1. Take your weight and multiply it by 10.

2. Take this number and multiply it by 0.5 and add it to the first number.

3. Now add in 100 calories for every mile you walk or run each day, or about 700 calories for every hour you exercise at a steady aerobic pace.

This number represents the amount of calories you need to eat each day to maintain the weight you are currently at under the exercise conditions you are undertaking.

Example:
160-lb. person who runs an average of three miles/day.
160 × 10 = 1,600
1600 × 0.5 = 800
800 + 1600 = 2,400
(3 miles) × 100 = 300
2400 + 300 = 2,700 calories per day to maintain current weight

If your interest is to lose weight, decrease your daily intake of this number by about 300 to 500 calories a day. This will result in a loss of about a pound of fat every seven to ten days. Never go below 1,200 calories daily, as this will trigger your body into starvation mode, causing you to hold on to every calorie you take in once you start eating at maintenance calorie levels.

This seemed to take my body composition even more toward the fat side, and I had stopped putting on muscle mass. One day, Brad, my strength coach, asked me what I ate. He said I had the perfect diet for a Sumo wrestler (a diet created to put on as much weight as possible). Starving during the day and bingeing at night slowed down my metabolism, and my starving body grabbed on to every calorie I ate. It's hard to get enough protein when

If you consume 100 calories a day more than your body needs, you will gain approximately ten pounds in a year. You could take that weight off, and keep it off, by doing thirty minutes of moderate exercise daily. The combination of exercise and diet offers the most flexible and effective approach to weight control.

you eat toast for breakfast and a cup of caffeine for lunch, no matter how big your dinner is.

Brad told me to eat five to six small meals a day (I had to eat something about every three hours), with each meal being no bigger than the palms of both hands held together. That is about the size of a small chicken breast, a half cup of rice and some veggies. He said that at least three of those meals should contain mostly protein. So I changed my portion size and eating frequency, and upped the protein.

At first, I felt as if I were overindulging in food by eating so frequently. It took some getting used to. But once I started to give my body food on a regular schedule, I found I was actually hungry every three hours. After the first week, my energy went up. My metabolism increased and the weight began to melt off. I know it was the change in my diet, because my workout load stayed the same. I also stopped craving carbohydrates and sugars at night.

I eventually realized that the only way to increase my metabolism was to give my body something to burn throughout the entire day. It finally made sense how Mark was able to eat all day long, even though he never ate much at any one sitting. It was an amazing experience to be eating instead of dieting to lose weight. I was pleasantly shocked.

The main things I try to do now are:

• Eat four to five small meals each day.

• Make sure just about every meal or snack has some protein in it.

• Stick with whole foods instead of supplements.

- Avoid empty calories.
- Take in foods that build me up instead of those that fill me up.

Counting Calories How can you look at a meal and have even the slightest clue what the calorie count is? If everything you eat comes from a box, the calories can be found by reading the labels. If you assemble your meals from fresh foods, the task may be a little more difficult.

Here are a few guidelines.

You can see that an 8-ounce serving of fish, chicken, or meat is going to be between 350 and 450 calories. A cup of carbohydrate or two slices of bread will add another 200 to 250. A salad with 3 tablespoons of oil-and-vinegar

CARBOHYDRATES	CALORIES	PROTEIN (G)	CARBOHYDRATES (G)	FAT (G)	FIBER (G)
Black beans	230/cup	15	40	1	15
Bread	90/slice	4	18	1.5	2
Couscous	200/cup	3.4	20.9	1	1.3
Corn	180/cup	5.5	41	2.2	4.6
Pasta	200/cup	13	80	2	5
Pinto beans	250/cup	14	43	8	15
Rice (brown)	300/cup	6	70	0	4

FRUIT AND VEGETABLES	CALORIES	PROTEIN (G)	CARBOHYDRATES (G)	FAT (G)	FIBER (G)
1 apple	70	0	18	0	6
1 banana	70	0	0	0	5
1 orange	70	0	0	0	5–6
All vegetables	around 50/cup				

PROTEINS	CALORIES	PROTEIN (G)	CARBOHYDRATES (G)	FAT (G)	FIBER (G)
Almonds	170/oz.	6	5	14	3
Beef, lean, 8 oz.	450	64	0	18	0
Chicken, no skin, 8 oz.	430	63	0	17	0
Cottage cheese, low fat (1%)	180/cup	28	8	2	0
Egg	75	6.3	6	5	0
Goat cheese, soft	75/oz.	5.3	.3	6	0
Milk, skim, 8 oz.	86	8	11.4	8.2	0
Mozzarella cheese, 1/2 cup shredded	160	14	2	12	0
Peanuts	159/oz.	7.2	4.5	13.8	2.5
Salmon, 8 oz.	320	50	0	13	0
Tofu	190/cup	10	2.3	5.9	1.5
Walnuts	172/oz.	7	3.4	16.1	1.4

FATS	CALORIES	PROTEIN(G)	CARBOHYDRATES(G)	FAT(G)	FIBER(G)
All oils	120/tsp.				
Butter	100/tbsp. (one stick is 4 oz. and about 800 cal.)				

dressing (mixed ⅓ water, ⅓ oil, ⅓ vinegar) will fill in an additional 120. A 2-ounce piece of cheese grated on top of the carbohydrate, or butter the two pieces of bread, and you have 200 more. The grand total: 400+200+120+200 = 920 calories. Add a low-fat yogurt for dessert and you are just over 1,050 for the meal. This is over one third of your total daily calorie intake in one sitting. If you have been eating several smaller meals throughout the day, this could be a problem. Eating one big meal late in the day is the ideal way to put on extra pounds. So this example—a fairly normal meal in most American homes—is a bit heavy for the last meal of the day.

Cut the protein serving down by one third and save 100 calories. Have one slice of bread or half a cup of carbohydrate and another 100 calories never reach the gullet. Hold the cheese or butter to 1 ounce and another 100 calories disappear out of the equation. Top the meal off with an apple instead of a yogurt for another 70-calorie savings and you are down to 680, or about one quarter of your daily intake instead of nearly half.

If you are on a high-carbohydrate diet and are exercising without seeing results in your body composition, add more protein and fat gradually, keeping track of what is happening in your body. Once you are satisfied after a meal, not searching for something else, then you have reached a dietary balance that is best for you.

Eating Smart Now comes phase two of smarter eating—getting the correct proportions of carbohydrates, proteins and fats. Not all calories are created equal in terms of optimizing your health. Let's take a look at a meal that gets roughly 40 percent of its calories from carbohydrates, 30 percent from protein, and 30 percent from fat.

First, balance the amount of carbohydrates and proteins you are eating. This will be the biggest step toward getting the right mix of calories for recovery and keeping your blood sugar stable.

The easiest way to do this is to look at your

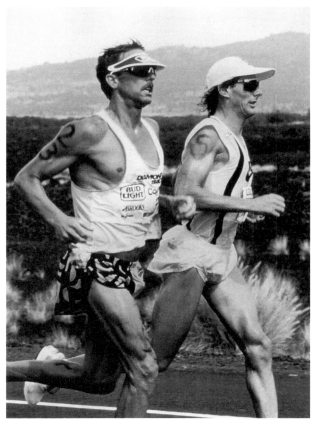

Running side by side with a guy like Dave Scott (left) was never fun. But to win the Ironman, I realized that I needed to have the courage to stay with the six-time champion all day long. We swam 2.4 miles, rode 112 miles, and ran over 24 miles together, never more than a few feet apart. In the last two miles, I finally surged away from him to win my first Ironman title. With that first one under my belt, the spell was broken: I went on to win in 1990, 1991, 1992, 1993, and 1995.

serving portions. The size of your protein portion should be about half the size of your carbohydrate. Keep in mind that the three pieces of bread you had before the main course are part of this equation. And if you must have dessert, try to eat one that has some protein along with it to balance the meal as a whole.

Next comes the fat. Look around your plate. If you can't see something with unsaturated or monounsaturated fats, try to add them in. Be aware that fats aren't always obvious. If you're eating animal proteins, there will always be some fat in the meat. The less meat you eat, however, the more important it is to include fat elsewhere in your diet. Sprinkle some olive oil over that pasta or add a dressing to the salad (one made from good oil instead of the creamy variety). Eat some walnuts or fish for the omega-3 oils and you're set. It's that simple.

As far as your daily intake goes, simply expand on the meal plan outlined above. Start by making sure there is enough protein in your diet. The average man requires about 55 grams of protein a day. That's about 8 ounces of meat and a cup of cottage cheese. If that same person is very active, the need for protein can double! From there, it's a matter of sizing your carbohydrate portions to be roughly twice the size of the protein portions and adding in some of all three types of fats, just as you do at each meal.

Mark: Mealtime Julie and I shop almost every day for the dinner food that night. This helps us tune in to what our bodies need to replenish and regenerate themselves. Even though a 40:30:30 (40 percent carbohydrates, 30 percent protein, 30 percent fat) diet is the ideal starting point, the exact ratio of carbohydrates, proteins, and fats that we need changes according to our training. Just like the difference in sleep needs from night to night, our food needs change also. It takes a little more effort, but the positives in health gains are more than worth it. And shopping for food and preparing meals has become quality family time at our house.

Julie: Cooking Together Mark and I have fun with food. He's a master of using condiments to spice up just about any meal. I'm better at coming up with something new that we've never had before. Fortunately, we both have an eye for healthy combinations. Together, we find ways to make dinner an adventure.

Basic Food Philosophy Eating healthily is a way of life, not a fourteen-day plan. Over time, we took the concepts of healthy eating and did our best to give them taste that kept us eating healthy meals because we actually *liked* them instead of out of duty to a dietary program.

We have a very Mediterranean diet. Olive oil, fresh herbs, fresh veggies, fish, poultry, freshly baked bread, and pasta make up the bulk of what we eat. Some Asian influences come from seasonings and the same fresh ingredients combined in a spicier way, then served with rice.

We love to experiment with new tastes, but our cupboards and freezer hold a basic stable of ingredients. The most in demand are olive oil (extra virgin, first-cold-pressing), fresh herbs—especially rosemary, cilantro, garlic, and onions—and some dried goodies like sun-dried tomatoes, both marinated and plain.

Our food philosophy boils down to the following basics:

• Read labels. If there are ingredients you have never heard of, your body probably won't like them.

• Limit starches. Choose between fresh-baked bread, pasta, or dessert, but not all three in one meal.

• Butter is better. Margarine is loaded with trans fats (partially hydrogenated fats), which cause a whole host of negative effects in your body.

• Choose nonfat. Whole fat milk, yogurt, and sour cream add extra saturated fats.

• Don't overcook rice, pasta, or other grains like oatmeal. Slightly undercooking these foods will slow their absorption, which translates into a lower glycemic (sugar) index.

• Buy organic from veggies to meats. The environment is far from being as clean as it was 100 years ago. Your body has to constantly filter out unnatural chemicals and compounds that enter your internal ecosystem through air, water, and food. If you can keep it clean in the areas within your control—such as the food you eat—your system will have to deal with fewer toxins overall.

• Reduce portion sizes and eat more slowly. The result will be eating less. You can eat a lot more quickly than you can absorb food into your bloodstream, which turns the appetite switch off. So go slowly and eat less. Think about how the food looks on the plate. While good presentation won't necessarily change the taste of food, it adds to the atmosphere and triggers that part of your brain that says the meal is something special, to be savored.

• Cook extra tonight with tomorrow's lunch in mind. Lunches can be the most difficult meal to be creative with. So, instead of having to come up with something in the morning on your way to work, just store the extras from the night before in individual-sized resealable containers for tomorrow's lunch.

• Every once in a while, go ahead and order the crème brûlée. Just split it with someone you love.

Basic Ingredients We try to have the basics on hand, so if time gets short and shopping is a stretch, there are always enough ingredients at home to throw something together at a moment's notice. Here are some of the staples we keep for emergencies:

In the refrigerator:

Butter

Canola oil (for cooking and baking)

Cheese (a little goes a long way)

Cilantro, basil, rosemary, green and white onions

Condiments (red chili paste, soy sauce, Dijon mustard, high-quality mayonnaise, rice wine vinegar, balsamic vinegar)

Corn tortillas

Eggs

Extra virgin, first-cold-pressing olive oil

Fresh fruit

Fresh pastas

Fruit-sweetened jams

Lemons and limes

Low-fat cream cheese

Nonfat milk

Nonfat yogurt

Nut butters

Salsa fresca

Spring mix for salads

Tomatoes

In the cupboard:

Canned organic beans—pinto, adzuki, white

Cereal

Dry pasta

Nuts—almonds, walnuts

Oats

Olives

Real maple syrup

Sun-dried tomatoes

Supplements—protein powder, electrolyte drinks, energy bars

Tuna

A Meal Plan We have provided a mix of meals that reflects our own eating habits and nutritional philosophy. The main part of each one is written out. Every meal is balanced for both calories and for a relatively healthy fat balance. However, they are not complete menus. If there is not enough food or variety in any one meal, just borrow some additional ideas from one of the other sections.

Breakfasts

POWER SHAKE: BREAKFAST IN A GLASS

2 scoops protein powder (vanilla or orange-flavored is the most versatile)

1 banana, frozen

½ cup water or nonfat milk

2 tablespoons flax seed oil

1 tablespoon nut butter (peanut, almond, or cashew)

Combine all the ingredients in a blender until smooth. Serves 1.

Tip: Using flavored yogurt instead of milk will increase the carbohydrate content, which is desirable if you are going to be working out shortly after drinking the shake.

POWER SHAKE NUTRITIONAL INFORMATION

Servings per recipe 1
Calories per serving 619
Cholesterol per serving (mg) 0

	Total grams	Percentage of total calories
Carbohydrates (1g=4Kcal)	63	39%
Protein (1g=4Kcal)	30	19%
Fat (1g=9Kcal)	30	42%

MARK'S FRENCH TOAST

1 whole egg plus 4 egg whites

2 slices whole grain bread

1 teaspoon canola oil

Nut butter (peanut, almond, or cashew)

Real maple syrup

Beat the eggs until smooth. Dip the bread into the beaten eggs. Grill in a lightly oiled skillet on both sides over medium-high heat until brown. Spread the nut butter on the French toast and spoon the syrup over the whole show. Serves 1.

Tip: Heating the maple syrup before pouring over the toast will enable you to use less. Spooning instead of pouring will also reduce the amount you use.

MARK'S FRENCH TOAST NUTRITIONAL INFORMATION

Servings per recipe 1
Calories per serving 435
Cholesterol per serving (mg) 242

	Total grams	Percentage of total calories
Carbohydrates (1g=4Kcal)	50	45%
Protein (1g=4Kcal)	27	25%
Fat (1g=9Kcal)	15	30%

LEFTOVER RICE "PANCAKES"

2 whole eggs plus 4 egg whites

1 cup leftover cooked white rice

1 teaspoon canola oil

½ cup plain low-fat yogurt

Real maple syrup

If you have rice left over from the night before, it can be used in place of the bread for the French toast recipe above. Simply use 2 whole eggs instead of 1 and add 1 cup of cooked leftover rice to the beaten eggs. Blend until all the rice is coated. Pour the entire mixture into a lightly oiled skillet over medium-high heat and spread flat like a pancake. Cook one side until golden brown, then flip (good luck!). If your cake comes apart at the seams, just scramble the whole mess in the pan until cooked through. It may not look pretty, but the taste is incredible. Spread with the yogurt and top with maple syrup. Serves 2.

LEFTOVER RICE "PANCAKES" NUTRITIONAL INFORMATION

Servings per recipe 2
Calories per serving 270
Cholesterol per serving (mg) 240

	Total grams	Percentage of total calories
Carbohydrates (1g=4Kcal)	54	42%
Protein (1g=4Kcal)	33	25%
Fat (1g=9Kcal)	19	33%

EGG BASICS

4 eggs

2 slices whole grain bread

Salt or salsa to taste

Bring to a boil a pot with enough water to cover the eggs. Drop the eggs in once the water is boiling and cook for 7 minutes. Toast the bread as the eggs are finishing up. Rinse the eggs with cold water, peel two of them, and put them on lightly buttered toast. Salt to taste or, for something a little spicier, add several teaspoons of salsa on top. Put the other two eggs in the refrigerator for another meal. Serves 2.

Tip: Eat with an apple, or have something citrus while the eggs are cooking, like an orange or grapefruit. Finish with a yogurt if you are still hungry.

EGG BASICS NUTRITIONAL INFORMATION

Servings per recipe 2
Calories per serving 397
Cholesterol per serving (mg) 489

	Total grams	Percentage of total calories
Carbohydrates (1g=4Kcal)	84	42%
Protein (1g=4Kcal)	41	21%
Fat (1g=9Kcal)	33	37%

EGG ADVANCED

THAI PEANUT SAUCE

¼ cup creamy peanut butter

Dash cayenne pepper

Splash soy sauce

2 tablespoons canned light coconut milk

2 to 3 tablespoons water

3 egg whites

¼ cup leftover cooked white rice

1 green onion, diced

1 Roma tomato, diced

½ cup leftover cooked broccoli, diced

Blend the sauce ingredients until smooth.

Cook the eggs as you would an omelet. (Pour eggs into a pan, cook until golden on one side, carefully flip and then cook the other side.) Place the remaining ingredients on top and fold over. Pour the peanut sauce on top. Serve with 1 slice whole wheat toast. Serves 1.

Tip: While the peanut sauce provides some fats, any leftover sauce will do. The eggs are just an excuse to have the sauce again.

EGG ADVANCED NUTRITIONAL INFORMATION

Servings per recipe	1	
Calories per serving	524	
Cholesterol per serving (mg)	7	
	Total grams	*Percentage of total calories*
Carbohydrates (1g=4Kcal)	57	42%
Protein (1g=4Kcal)	32	23%
Fat (1g=9Kcal)	21	35%

EGG FINALE

1 whole egg plus 1 egg white

½ cup of any of the following: cooked turkey sausage, leftover cooked chicken, tofu, cottage cheese, or just about any protein you can think of

2 slices whole grain toast, buttered

In a skillet over medium-high heat, scramble the eggs. Heat the other protein source. Scoop onto the toast or just eat alongside. Serves 1.

Tip: This is a high-protein breakfast that takes less than 5 minutes to assemble and cook. As with any of the breakfasts, if you feel the need for something sweet, finish with a flavored yogurt or an apple, or start with a citrus fruit.

EGG FINALE NUTRITIONAL INFORMATION

Servings per recipe	1	
Calories per serving	487	
Cholesterol per serving (mg)	266	
	Total grams	*Percentage of total calories*
Carbohydrates (1g=4Kcal)	54	44%
Protein (1g=4Kcal)	33	27%
Fat (1g=9Kcal)	16	29%

BEANS AND TORTILLAS

½ cup cooked or canned pinto or black beans, drained

2 corn tortillas

¼ avocado, sliced

Salsa to taste

Fresh cilantro

Heat the beans in one half of a skillet. In the other half, heat the tortillas on both sides. Put the tortillas on a plate. Scoop the beans on top. Add the sliced avocado, salsa, and cilantro. Roll up and dive in. Serves 1.

Tip: This is the original complete-protein meal of beans and corn. You get a complete protein as well as omega-3 fats from the beans, plus a lot of fiber. If you think it's boring, try a different salsa. Add 3 ounces of skinless roasted chicken for an almost perfect 40:30:30 meal.

BEANS AND TORTILLAS NUTRITIONAL INFORMATION

Servings per recipe	1	
Calories per serving	498	
Cholesterol per serving (mg)	72	
	Total grams	*Percentage of total calories*
Carbohydrates (1g=4Kcal)	50	40%
Protein (1g=4Kcal)	36	29%
Fat (1g=9Kcal)	17	31%

Lunches

ALBACORE TUNA SANDWICH

One 6-ounce can water-packed white-meat or albacore tuna, drained

2 tablespoons sweet pickle relish

1 stalk celery, chopped

1 carrot, grated

2 tablespoons mayonnaise or ¼ avocado, diced

2 slices whole grain bread

In a medium bowl, combine all the ingredients except the bread. Spread onto one slice of the bread, topping with the remaining slice. Serves 1.

Tip: Scoop the tuna mixture onto any kind of flatbread crackers instead of making a traditional sandwich. This keeps the meal a little lighter. Assemble it at work or school, too—just put crackers in a baggie and bring the tuna in a sealed container. Finally, an end to the soggy sammy.

ALBACORE TUNA SANDWICH NUTRITIONAL INFORMATION		
Servings per recipe	1	
Calories per serving	499	
Cholesterol per serving (mg)	71	
	Total grams	Percentage of total calories
Carbohydrates (1g=4Kcal)	18	39%
Protein (1g=4Kcal)	41	33%
Fat (1g=9Kcal)	14	28%

EGG SALAD SANDWICH

2 hard-boiled eggs plus 3 hard-boiled egg whites

2 tablespoons sweet pickle relish

1 stalk celery, chopped

1 carrot, grated

2 tablespoons mayonnaise or ¼ avocado, diced

2 slices whole grain bread

Remember those leftover eggs that you cooked yesterday for breakfast? Break them out, peel and chop them, then combine with the remaining ingredients, except the bread. The inside for your sandwich—or the topping for flatbread crackers—is ready to go. Spoon filling onto one slice of the bread and top with the remaining slice. Serves 1.

Tip: An apple, a handful of almonds, or ½ cup of cottage cheese is a good addition if you are still hungry. Just keep in mind that apples are carbohydrates, and the other options are protein. Which is your body calling out for more of today?

EGG SALAD SANDWICH NUTRITIONAL INFORMATION		
Servings per recipe	1	
Calories per serving	490	
Cholesterol per serving (mg)	483	
	Total grams	Percentage of total calories
Carbohydrates (1g=4Kcal)	48	40%
Protein (1g=4Kcal)	30	25%
Fat (1g=9Kcal)	19	35%

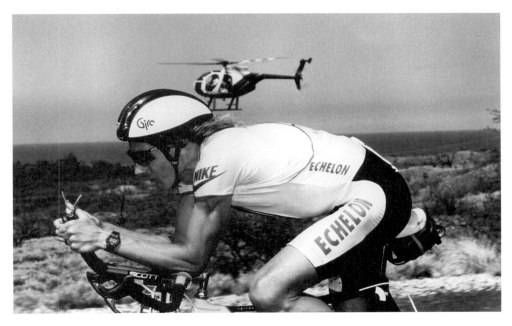

Sometimes being in the spotlight makes it tough to just zone out and race your own race. Having a helicopter hovering over you all day long can be a tad disconcerting.

QUESADILLAS

2 corn tortillas

½ cup cooked or canned beans, or any leftover protein

Salsa or chopped tomatoes

Fresh cilantro

Shredded cheese (optional)

Heat the tortillas in one half of a skillet. In the other half, heat the beans or protein. Scoop the beans onto the tortillas and garnish with the rest of the ingredients. Serves 1.

Tip: This looks a lot like the Beans and Tortillas breakfast (page 126). Well, it is. The only real difference is that you are eating it at lunch and not in the morning.

QUESADILLAS NUTRITIONAL INFORMATION

Servings per recipe	1	
Calories per serving	572	
Cholesterol per serving (mg)	0	
	Total grams	Percentage of total calories
Carbohydrates (1g=4Kcal)	57	41%
Protein (1g=4Kcal)	42	30%
Fat (1g=9Kcal)	18	29%

SALAD AS A MEAL

DRESSING

¼ cup olive oil

¼ cup balsamic vinegar

2 tablespoons water

1 tablespoon Dijon mustard

2 tablespoons soy sauce or to taste

4 cups organic greens

Sliced organic veggies of your choice

Leftover cooked salmon, chicken, hummus, or cottage cheese

Flatbread crackers (optional)

Combine the dressing ingredients and mix until thoroughly blended. In a separate bowl, combine the greens, veggies, and salmon or chicken. (If using hummus or cottage cheese, do *not* add them yet.) Add the dressing and toss. Eat with crackers if you included salmon or chicken in the salad or with crackers and hummus or cottage cheese if no animal protein is used in the salad. Serves 2.

Tip: As with any salad, using extra virgin olive oil in the dressing is a great way to get a good share of your daily need for monounsaturated fats.

SALAD AS A MEAL NUTRITIONAL INFORMATION

Servings per recipe	2	
Calories per serving	412	
Cholesterol per serving (mg)	varies	
	Total grams	Percentage of total calories
Carbohydrates (1g=4Kcal)	71	39%
Protein (1g=4Kcal)	54	29%
Fat (1g=9Kcal)	26	32%

MORE BASIC THAN BASIC: PB&J

2 slices whole grain bread

2 tablespoons peanut butter

1 tablespoon spreadable fruit

You can probably figure out what to do with this one. Take the bread and add the peanut butter and the spreadable fruit. Top it off with a yogurt, or some cottage cheese and an apple. Serves 1.

Tip: PB&J is a good standby when the creative cook is on leave. This meal may sound like kids-only, but it's actually a great balance of carbohydrates, fats, and proteins.

MORE BASIC THAN BASIC: PB&J NUTRITIONAL INFORMATION

Servings per recipe	1	
Calories per serving	445	
Cholesterol per serving (mg)	9	
	Total grams	Percentage of total calories
Carbohydrates (1g=4Kcal)	45	40%
Protein (1g=4Kcal)	28	24%
Fat (1g=9Kcal)	18	36%

Leftover Madness

Remember those leftovers from last night? If they were packed in individual-sized containers, it's simply a matter of pulling them out and gobbling them down. There's no preparation time, other than maybe a little re-heating. We don't cook with the microwave, but will use it for some of the leftovers.

Dinners

NOT-JUST-FOR-VEGETARIANS VEGGIE WALNUT-PARSLEY PASTA

½ cup chopped walnuts

¼ cup grated Parmesan cheese

½ cup chopped fresh parsley

3 tablespoons chopped fresh sage

3 tablespoons chopped fresh chives

2 tablespoons minced garlic

2 tablespoons olive oil

1 cup vegetable broth

Splash white wine (optional)

Salt to taste

12 ounces fresh uncooked pasta

Combine the walnuts, Parmesan, and fresh herbs in a bowl and set aside. Sauté the garlic in the olive oil. Add the broth and wine. Simmer uncovered to cook off the alcohol. Season with salt. Meanwhile, cook the pasta in boiling water until al dente. Rinse, then combine with hot garlic mixture. Stir in the herb mixture and serve immediately. Serves 3.

Tip: This pasta takes about as long to cook as it takes to boil a pot of water for the noodles. Add a side of salmon or serve cottage cheese over a salad and you have a perfectly balanced meal that tastes great.

Veggie Walnut-Parsley Pasta Nutritional Information		
Servings per recipe	3	
Calories per serving	714	
Cholesterol per serving (mg)	124	
	Total grams	Percentage of total calories
Carbohydrates (1g=4Kcal)	221	41%
Protein (1g=4Kcal)	130	24%
Fat (1g=9Kcal)	83	35%

SEA BASS WITH CILANTRO-GINGER SAUCE

1 clove garlic

½ jalapeño chili pepper (wash hands and cutting surface well after using)

1 tablespoon fresh ginger, peeled and chopped

Saturday Night

Not every night is reserved for the healthiest meal in the shortest amount of time. We usually like to keep Saturday night open for entertaining friends. Our staple party dinner used to be lasagna or a layered Mexican casserole. However, now our taste has lightened up, and we serve something grilled with a sauce, a side of rice or pasta, and a salad. Dessert is tea and maybe a fruit sorbet served by the fire in winter, or fresh fruit in summer. Mark makes a great pumpkin pie and Julie can be talked into a fresh fruit cobbler on a really special occasion. But generally, our guests don't expect dessert, especially when we offer larger main-course portions.

Juice of 2 limes

1 bunch fresh cilantro, coarsely chopped

¼ cup olive oil

Salt and pepper to taste

1½ pounds or 4 pieces sea bass, fresh if possible

Hot cooked rice or soba noodles

Put the first five ingredients in a blender. Turn on low and slowly drizzle in the olive oil. Blend until the sauce is bright green and smooth. Season with salt and pepper.

Season the sea bass with salt and pepper. Brush the top of each piece with some of the sauce.

Fill a deep heavy skillet with about 1 inch of water and bring to a boil. Place a steamer basket in the skillet and place the fish in the basket. Cover and steam 5 to 6 minutes, or until fish is just cooked through. Remove and serve over rice or soba noodles. Spoon additional sauce over the top. Serves 4.

Tip: Any white fish works with this recipe. Also, try doubling the sauce recipe. By making extra, there will be leftovers to spoon over just about anything that needs a little help waking up its natural flavor. If you have friends coming who don't eat fish, simply boil some pasta for them and top with a healthy handful of pine nuts, ¼ cup cooked pinto or adzuki beans, and several scoops of the cilantro-ginger sauce.

Sea Bass with Cilantro-Ginger Sauce Nutritional Information

Servings per recipe	4	
Calories per serving	643	
Cholesterol per serving (mg)	42	
	Total grams	Percentage of total calories
Carbohydrates (1g=4Kcal)	270	43%
Protein (1g=4Kcal)	180	28%
Fat (1g=9Kcal)	82	29%

CHICKEN WITH ORANGE-BASIL-MINT PESTO

1 cup packed fresh basil leaves

1 cup packed fresh mint leaves

½ cup shelled walnuts

2 cloves garlic

¼ cup fresh orange juice

¼ cup olive oil

Salt and pepper to taste

2 whole boneless, skinless chicken breasts

Hot cooked couscous or rice

In a blender or food processor, combine the first four ingredients until well blended, adding orange juice to taste. With the machine still going, drizzle in the olive oil and blend until smooth. You can add a little extra if it is still too dry. Season with salt and pepper.

Grill one side of the chicken breasts until golden. Flip the breasts and scoop a spoonful of pesto onto them. Continue grilling until done. Serve over couscous or rice. Add additional sauce to taste. Serves 4.

Tip: This dish can be turned into a mouthwatering vegetarian meal by replacing each person's chicken breast portion with a cup of cooked Northern white beans and serving it over couscous with a topping of the pesto. Complete the meal with a vegetable like artichokes.

Chicken with Orange-Basil-Mint Pesto Nutritional Information

Servings per recipe	4	
Calories per serving	680	
Cholesterol per serving (mg)	10	
	Total grams	Percentage of total calories
Carbohydrates (1g=4Kcal)	242	36%
Protein (1g=4Kcal)	194	29%
Fat (1g=9Kcal)	108	35%

GRILLED SIRLOIN STEAKS WITH TARRAGON-GARLIC BUTTER

¼ cup white wine

2 tablespoons chopped shallots

¼ teaspoon dried tarragon

3 tablespoons butter, at room temperature

1 clove garlic, minced

¼ cup toasted walnut pieces

1 tablespoon chopped fresh tarragon

Salt and pepper to taste

2 sirloin steaks

Steamed vegetables

4 cups salad

2 cups yellow and red pepper strips

4 pita breads

1 cup hummus

Boil the wine, shallots, and dried tarragon until the liquid evaporates, forming a paste. Don't overcook. Let cool to room temperature. Add the butter, garlic, walnut pieces, and chopped fresh tarragon to the mixture. Season with salt and pepper. On a sheet of waxed paper, form the mixture into a log and refrigerate.

Season the steaks with salt and pepper. Let stand until room temperature. Grill the steaks until desired doneness, about 5 minutes per side for medium well. Remove from the heat and let stand for 5 minutes to seal in the juices. Top each steak with a teaspoon of the butter mixture. Serve with steamed vegetables of your choice, tossed salad with pepper strips, and pita with hummus. Serves 4.

Tip: This has the potential to be quite a heavy meal. Remember that a little of the butter will go a long way. The meal will be more digestible if you have your main carbohydrates as an appetizer. Then, with the steak, limit your carbohydrate intake. Fill the dinner plate and your tummy up with additional vegetables instead of potatoes or bread. Instead of dessert, finish the meal off with a flavored tea, such as licorice. It's naturally sweet and can satisfy that urge for sugar.

Grilled Sirloin Steaks with Tarragon-Garlic Butter
Nutritional Information

	Total grams	Percentage of total calories
Servings per recipe	4	
Calories per serving	682	
Cholesterol per serving (mg)	131	
Carbohydrates (1g=4Kcal)	60	36%
Protein (1g=4Kcal)	46	28%
Fat (1g=9Kcal)	24	36%

GRILLED SALMON WITH THAI MARINADE

½ cup rice wine vinegar

½ cup fresh lime juice

¼ cup toasted sesame oil

⅛ cup canola oil

⅛ cup olive oil

1 pound salmon steaks or fillets

Salt and pepper to taste

Lime wedges

4 cups hot cooked rice

Mix the vinegar, lime juice, sesame oil, canola oil, and olive oil in a small bowl.

Place the fish in a large glass baking dish. Pour the marinade over the salmon. Season with salt and pepper. Cover and chill for 2 to 3 hours. (If there is not enough time to marinate the salmon, just get the grill going and start cooking, saving a small amount of the marinade to pour over the salmon once it has been flipped to cook the second side.)

Heat the grill. Place the salmon on, skin side down. Grill approximately 5 to 7 minutes or until the uncooked side is opaque. Flip and grill the other side for about half the time of the first side. Serve with lime wedges over rice with a side of citrus salad. Serves 4.

Tip: This marinade works great for tofu stir-fry. Brown strips of tofu in a hot skillet, add a blend of your favorite diced veggies, and cook until tender. Drizzle the marinade over the mixture to taste once cooking is complete. To bring in even more of the Thai influence, add a few dashes of cayenne pepper to the marinade. Serve over rice or noodles.

Grilled Salmon with Thai Marinade Nutritional Information

	Total grams	Percentage of total calories
Servings per recipe	4	
Calories per serving	556	
Cholesterol per serving (mg)	70	
Carbohydrates (1g=4Kcal)	200	35%
Protein (1g=4Kcal)	158	28%
Fat (1g=9Kcal)	10	37%

CHILI-STUFFED SWEET POTATOES

4 large sweet potatoes

1 tablespoon olive oil

1 cup diced green bell peppers

1 cup diced yellow bell peppers

1½ cups chopped white onions

1 tablespoon minced garlic

1 tablespoon chili powder

2 teaspoons ground cumin

1 16 ounce can diced and peeled tomatoes with juice

1 16 ounce can black beans, rinsed

2 cups diced and drained squash of your choice

1 tablespoon finely minced seeded jalapeño chilies

Lime wedges and fresh cilantro

Plain nonfat yogurt for topping

Preheat the oven to 400 degrees. Place the potatoes in a baking dish. Pierce with a fork and bake until tender, about 1 to 1½ hours.

While the potatoes are baking, heat the olive oil in a large skillet over medium-high heat. Add the bell peppers and onions; sauté until lightly browned. Add the garlic and cook until tender. Next add the chili powder and cumin, then the tomatoes and beans. Reduce the heat and simmer for 20 minutes. Add the squash and jalapeños. Cover the skillet and cook until the squash is just done, about 5 minutes.

Place the potatoes on individual plates. Split them and scoop the chili onto the center of each one. Squeeze lime juice over them. Top with cilantro and yogurt. Serves 4.

Tip: Chili leftovers make a great lunch the next day. For variety, serve over rice or even toast.

Anytime beans are combined with a grain, you have a complete protein.

CHILI-STUFFED SWEET POTATOES NUTRITIONAL INFORMATION

		Percentage of
Servings per recipe	4	
Calories per serving	656	
Cholesterol per serving (mg)	42	
	Total grams	total calories
Carbohydrates (1g=4Kcal)	294	44%
Protein (1g=4Kcal)	222	34%
Fat (1g=9Kcal)	8	22%

SATURDAY NITE CHICKEN

1 tablespoon ginger, chopped

1 tablespoon turmeric

1 tablespoon curry powder

¼ cup chopped fresh mint

2 cups chicken broth

1 cup canned coconut milk

1 cup plain nonfat yogurt

3 pounds boneless, skinless chicken breast, cut into small cubes

2 tablespoons olive oil

¼ cup lime juice

TOPPERS

1 banana, peeled and sliced

1 apple, cored and chopped

2 medium bell peppers, chopped

½ cup golden raisins

¼ cup mandarin slices

½ cup peanuts

3 green onions, chopped

Heat the olive oil in a pot over medium heat. Sauté the onions in the oil. Add the ginger, curry powder, turmeric, and mint. Sauté about a minute. Add the yogurt and cook for 1 minute, stirring constantly. Add the lime juice and chicken broth and bring to a boil. Reduce heat and simmer until the sauce starts to thicken, stirring regularly, about 30 minutes.

Cook the chicken in a skillet until the juice runs clear, then add it to the pot along with the coconut milk. Simmer about 10 minutes, then serve over Spicy Rice (recipe follows). Place each of the toppers in a separate bowl and pass at the table to accompany the curry as desired. Serves 6.

Tip: This is the most labor-intensive of our dishes, but it's worth the time it takes. This is easily converted to a high-protein vegetarian meal by replacing the chicken with tofu, which should be cubed and browned, and substituting a vegetable stock for the chicken broth. Either way, it's guaranteed to please.

SPICY RICE

2 cups uncooked basmati rice

2 bay leaves

2 sticks cinnamon

4 cups cold water

Place all the ingredients in a pot and bring to a boil, then lower the heat and simmer until the rice is done and all the water is absorbed, about 20 minutes.

SATURDAY NITE CHICKEN WITH SPICY RICE NUTRITIONAL INFORMATION

		Percentage of
Servings per recipe	6	
Calories per serving	979	
Cholesterol per serving (mg)	10	
	Total grams	total calories
Carbohydrates (1g=4Kcal)	567	39%
Protein (1g=4Kcal)	511	35%
Fat (1g=9Kcal)	169	26%

Salads, Sauces, and Sides

CITRUS SALAD

2 tablespoons fresh grapefruit juice (can also use tangerine juice)

1 tablespoon white wine vinegar

¼ cup olive oil

Salt and pepper to taste

Vegetables (red or yellow cherry tomatoes, red onion, grated carrots, and bell pepper all go well)

1 package fresh organic spring mix

1 bunch arugula, optional

1 can mandarin oranges

¾ cup lowfat cottage cheese

Mix the first four ingredients until smooth. In a serving dish, add your favorite veggies to the greens. Add the mandarin oranges to accent the citrus dressing. Pour the dressing over the salad and serve with the cottage cheese. Serves 3.

CITRUS SALAD NUTRITIONAL INFORMATION		
Servings per recipe	3	
Calories per serving	244	
Cholesterol per serving (mg)	5	
	Total grams	Percentage of total calories
Carbohydrates (1g=4Kcal)	74	40%
Protein (1g=4Kcal)	48	26%
Fat (1g=9Kcal)	58	34%

NOT YOUR MOM'S COLESLAW

DRESSING

6 tablespoons rice wine vinegar

3 tablespoons canola oil

5 tablespoons creamy peanut butter

3 tablespoons soy sauce

3 tablespoons golden brown sugar

2 tablespoons minced fresh ginger

1½ tablespoons minced garlic

1 cup thinly sliced bok choy, arugula, or spinach

3 cups thinly sliced green cabbage

2 cups thinly sliced red cabbage

1 large yellow bell pepper, sliced into very thin strips

1 large red bell pepper, sliced into very thin strips

2 medium carrots, sliced into thin strips

3 green onions, thinly sliced

½ cup chopped fresh cilantro

Salt and pepper to taste

Mix the dressing ingredients in a small bowl. This can be made ahead and refrigerated. Combine the remaining ingredients except the salt and pepper in a large bowl. Add the dressing and toss to coat. Season with salt and pepper. Add a serving of boiled or steamed shrimp for a complete meal. Serves 6.

NOT YOUR MOM'S COLESLAW NUTRITIONAL INFORMATION		
Servings per recipe	6	
Calories per serving	312	
Cholesterol per serving (mg)	148	
	Total grams	Percentage of total calories
Carbohydrates (1g=4Kcal)	174	35%
Protein (1g=4Kcal)	137	28%
Fat (1g=9Kcal)	81	37%

Meals on Wheels

Sometimes you know you will be somewhere that is just not good for carrying either leftovers or a fresh lunch. This is when some other options are needed. Here are two possibilities:

OPTION ONE: Energy bars. Have several energy bars that are composed of calories of roughly 40:30:30. These fit inside any briefcase, purse, or backpack and can be eaten anywhere, anytime.

OPTION TWO: Nuts and fruit. Our favorite road snack is tamari-roasted almonds and apples. Have a baggie with almonds ready to go. Bring an apple to eat with it. The almonds provide a good source of protein and some good oils. The apple lends a little carbohydrate in a slowly absorbable form. The combination of salty from the tamari and sweet from the apple seems to satisfy both of those urges.

Regardless of which option you choose, both will definitely hold off the urge to stop in at your local fast-food joint and grab something that you will probably regret eating later.

ROSEMARY POTATO SALAD

2½ pounds red potatoes, unpeeled and cut into wedges

6 tablespoons olive oil

¼ cup fresh lemon juice

1 teaspoon lemon zest

2 tablespoons drained capers

2 tablespoons chopped fresh rosemary

1½ teaspoons minced garlic

Salt and pepper to taste

Cook the potatoes in a pot of boiling salted water until just done. Drain and let the potatoes cool.

Mix the olive oil, lemon juice, zest, capers, rosemary, and garlic together. Season with salt and pepper. Pour the dressing over warm, not hot, potatoes. Toss to coat. Serve warm or chilled. Add a serving of boneless, skinless chicken for a complete meal. Serves 4.

ROSEMARY POTATO SALAD NUTRITIONAL INFORMATION		
Servings per recipe	4	
Calories per serving	637	
Cholesterol per serving (mg)	0	
	Total grams	Percentage of total calories
Carbohydrates (1g=4Kcal)	245	38%
Protein (1g=4Kcal)	165	26%
Fat (1g=9Kcal)	102	36%

LEMON SPINACH WITH OLIVE OIL

½ package fresh spinach leaves (about 2 cups)

2 tablespoons olive oil

2 tablespoons fresh lemon juice

Salt to taste

Heat ⅓ cup water in a large pot until just boiling. Add the spinach in batches. Cook until just wilted. Drain the spinach and place in a serving dish. Add the olive oil and lemon juice. Season with salt. Toss and serve warm on the top of sliced Italian chiabatta bread. An 8-ounce serving of nonfat yogurt completes the meal. Serves 2.

LEMON SPINACH WITH OLIVE OIL NUTRITIONAL INFORMATION		
Servings per recipe	2	
Calories per serving	184	
Cholesterol per serving (mg)	0	
	Total grams	Percentage of total calories
Carbohydrates (1g=4Kcal)	40	40%
Protein (1g=4Kcal)	21	21%
Fat (1g=9Kcal)	16	39%

STEAMED ARTICHOKES

2 artichokes

Lemon wedges

Olive oil

Cut off the top third of the artichoke leaves before steaming. Place the artichokes in a steamer and cook until a fork inserted in the heart of the artichoke goes in easily. Remove from the steamer and drizzle lemon juice over the artichokes. To eat, remove leaves and dip in olive oil. Add broiled or baked salmon and a French baguette for a delicious, complete meal. Serves 2.

STEAMED ARTICHOKES NUTRITIONAL INFORMATION		
Servings per recipe	2	
Calories per serving	80	
Cholesterol per serving (mg)	0	
	Total grams	Percentage of total calories
Carbohydrates (1g=4Kcal)	98	39%
Protein (1g=4Kcal)	84	33%
Fat (1g=9Kcal)	32	28%

CAN'T STOP HUMMUS

2 16-ounce cans Great Northern white beans, rinsed

1 tablespoon chopped garlic

⅓ cup fresh lemon juice

¼ cup tahini

¼ cup olive oil

Salt and pepper to taste

3 tablespoons chopped fresh mint

¼ cup finely chopped fresh parsley

Place the beans along with the garlic in a food processor fitted with a steel blade. Process until just combined. Add the lemon juice, tahini, and olive oil. Blend until smooth. Add a bit of water if the mixture is too thick. Season with salt and pepper. Transfer to a small bowl. Add the mint and parsley just before serving. Serve on pita bread or veggies. It's so good you can't stop eating it! Add a portion of nonfat Cheddar cheese to get the protein you need. Serves 4.

CAN'T STOP HUMMUS NUTRITIONAL INFORMATION		
Servings per recipe	4	
Calories per serving	421	
Cholesterol per serving (mg)	38	
	Total grams	Percentage of total calories
Carbohydrates (1g=4Kcal)	174	39%
Protein (1g=4Kcal)	125	28%
Fat (1g=9Kcal)	63	32%

GREEN OLIVE SPREAD (TAPENADE)

1 cup chopped pitted green olives

½ cup chopped walnuts

½ cup chopped fresh parsley

¼ cup chopped fresh arugula

½ cup chopped white onions

⅓ cup olive oil

3 tablespoons fresh lemon juice

¼ teaspoon dried crushed red peppers

1 teaspoon lemon zest

Salt and pepper to taste

Combine all the ingredients except the salt and pepper in a food processor fitted with a steel blade. Using the on/off button for quick pulses, mix just until olive spread holds together (do not overmix). Place in a bowl and season to taste with salt and pepper. Serve with fresh bread and veggies like fresh sliced carrots, celery, and bell pepper. Add a pound of boiled or steamed shrimp for protein. Serves 4.

GREEN OLIVE SPREAD (TAPENADE) NUTRITIONAL INFORMATION		
Servings per recipe	4	
Calories per serving	412	
Cholesterol per serving (mg)	221	
	Total grams	Percentage of total calories
Carbohydrates (1g=4Kcal)	131	31%
Protein (1g=4Kcal)	130	31%
Fat (1g=9Kcal)	76	38%

Share the Mood, Not the Food An occasional celebration with something decadent is quite acceptable. The problem is that it can seem like the world is conspiring to keep you forever gorging on everything but the healthy stuff. Think about all the food that passes through an office during the course of a week.

On Monday, it's leftover sweets from Sam's in-laws. Tuesday is Clare's big fiftieth birthday, and of course she loves (and expects) double-rich flourless chocolate cake. Wednesday is the usual midweek office meeting, where someone invariably brings something decadent in hopes of softening the blow of yet another deadline that no one expected. By Thursday, you're thinking it

couldn't continue, but it does. Andy closes the deal of his life, and to thank all of you who helped, he brings in a box of imported Swiss chocolates to show his gratitude.

Wow! Chocolate twice in one week! Then TGIF, no suits, a company lunch of processed-cheesy nachos and grease-soaked deep-fried chimichangas, and olé! It's time for the weekend sports parties parked in front of the tube for hours on end with beer and buttery popcorn. On top of all this are the three to five small meals that you should be eating each day.

How can you possibly say no to some or all of these undoubtedly delicious extras without offending every coworker and rich relative on the planet?

Realize that food is often the vehicle for bringing people together to share a common sense of celebration and closeness. Be a part of that atmosphere in mood and presence without stuffing something in your mouth that you won't feel good about later. Don't make a big deal about turning down an offer to scarf down a slab of something you don't want. A simple "It does look really delicious, but I'm fine for now" will do.

Share in the celebration, but remember that, ultimately, feeling happy about yourself comes from being healthy and active and from choosing a diet that supports those goals. When it's your turn to bring in the goodies, make it delicious *and* healthy (yes, the two can go hand in hand).

Snacks Here is a Top 10 list of snacks to fill in the gaps between meals. Try always to include some protein, even in a snack. It keeps you from grabbing the quick-fix "treats" that are all too easy to eat and so hard to burn off.

1. String cheese and half a bagel
2. 40:30:30 nutrition bars
3. Low-fat or nonfat yogurt
4. A hard-boiled egg and crackers
5. Cottage cheese and apple slices
6. Hummus and pita slices
7. Almonds

8. A meal-replacement drink

9. Bowl of whole grain cereal (so it's not breakfast . . . who's looking?)

10. Leftover anything from the night before (sounds boring, but it's better than a doughnut or a bag of fries)

I Blew It Again What happens when you try to eat healthy and one day you find yourself back at Mrs. Fields having a big chocolate-chip cookie? If you judge the entire program on that one moment, you may feel like a failure. Depressed and angry with yourself, you might decide this proper diet stuff is just too hard.

We all have weak moments when we cave in. If you judge the entire program at your weakest moments, it will look pretty futile. But one slide into the dessert section of the grocery store does not constitute a failure. One chocolate binge after a bad day at the office isn't the end of the world. In fact, reaching short-term goals of fitness, regularity of workouts, body composition changes, or weight loss or gain could be the perfect time to consciously reward yourself with something on the banned list. Remember, it's what you do *most of the time* that counts.

Nutrition and Kids Explaining to your child why some foods are healthy and why some are not will at least give him a base of knowledge that will be rumbling around in their heads every time they want to trade their apple slices for a Snickers bar. Beyond that, don't expect them to exhibit any behavior other than what they see consistently at home. If you eat smart and avoid being obsessive about food, they will do the same. If you consistently sneak and splurge, expect them to pick up on that as well.

We talk a lot with Mats about what is in different foods. He still loves junk, but will actually make, on his own, healthy choices most of the time.

When blood sugar is low, the brain wants to bring it up quickly. Avoiding this is the best guard against the good food giveaway. If the jewel of your life has low blood sugar and is

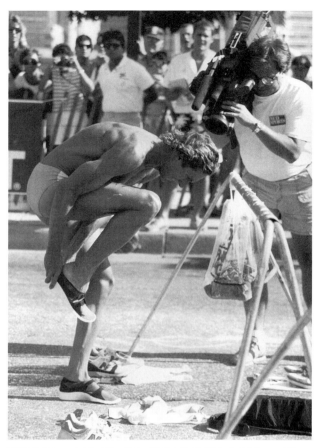

This time I was lucky enough to find the right transition spot. Once, the camera followed me in as I struggled for what seemed like an eternity before I realized that I was in the wrong parking spot trying to squeeze into someone's way-too-small shoes!

faced with a lunchbox filled with cold pasta and a stinky piece of salmon, you know she is going to grab someone's Yoo-hoos or Ding-Dongs! Instead, give her a good breakfast—whole wheat toast with butter, a poached egg with some avocado, and an apple—then send her out the door full.

Eating a healthy breakfast is one of the best things you and your child can do to jump-start your bodies into a healthy state for the day. Skipping breakfast or having one made up of cinnamon buns sets your internal balancing act up for the insulin joyride. If Junior leaves with a bowl of Sugar Crunch Nuggets in his little tummy, there will inevitably be a time later when his brain calls out for more, and the auction for junk food begins.

School Lunches The best thing is to make a little bit extra every night for dinner and put some of it aside for lunch the next day. If you are making enchiladas, make a few for Junior's lunch. If you make some pasta with chicken, put some aside in a container that seals tightly. If your child liked the dinner, then leftovers for lunch will probably be a bigger hit than the same sandwich he has had every day for the past three weeks.

Nutrition Nuggets

- Get most of your carbohydrates from complex forms. Put (very) simply, sugar is a simple carbohydrate. Whole grain is a complex one.

- Monitor your body's response to gray-area carbohydrates like white pasta. Feeling sleepy, sluggish, or bloated after eating is a sign to stick with complex carbohydrates.

- Avoid simple carbohydrates such as refined sugars and grains.

- Eat a balance of fats and oils (unsaturated, monounsaturated, saturated).

- Avoid fried foods (they cause fats to become rancid) and partially hydrogenated fats.

- Protein portions should be roughly half the size of your carbohydrate portion.

- Eat four to six smaller meals throughout the day, making sure to include enough protein.

- Savor the meal and stop eating before you are stuffed. It takes a while for the food that is eaten to be absorbed into your bloodstream and turn off your appetite-control mechanism.

- Substitute fresh foods for processed foods, and drink enough liquids throughout the day. Being dehydrated can actually be confused with being hungry.

- Try to replenish lost liquids and nutrients within a half hour of ending your workouts.

11 Kid Fitness

Kids love to run—always have, always will. Capture the flag, freeze tag, pickle, red rover, hide-and-seek, kick the can . . . these are all games that kids naturally take to. They giggle and smile ear to ear as they scurry around the neighborhood with their buddies. They don't realize or care that they are developing cardiovascular fitness, but they are.

Somewhere along the line, a fitness instructor at school starts to use running as punishment. You're late to line up for PE, so you have to run a lap. Your team lost in basketball, so you have to run a lap. The enjoyment that kids naturally derive from running can disappear in a flash. Running is no longer a natural, fun experience. It is to be avoided, a penance for crimes against the coach, a drag.

That's why it is so important to remember that fitness should always be fun. Your children aren't working out, they are *playing*. There is a huge difference between the two. It's not a bad idea to keep that fun factor alive in *your* life as well. Make sure you look at your fitness activities as a reprieve from the mundane, as an escape from work. You'll enjoy your fitness activities 100 percent more.

Mats: Fun It's most important to have fun. That's the most important thing when you are running or swimming or biking. I don't really know if my friends like to do all these things. But I do.

Mark: Running with Mats Mats already has the fitness bug. Since Julie and I both love to run, Mats loves to run. We will go out after one of our own runs and cruise through the neighborhood with Mats, chatting and joking and having a good time. Sometimes he runs as far as a mile, but the distance and pace are irrelevant. Our family runs have become a special time for all three of us.

When Mats was younger, Julie used to run and push the Baby Jogger with Mats in it. In fact, she'll tell you that those workouts pushing an extra fifty pounds of kid and ten pounds of Baby Jogger were a huge help to her as she got ready for the New York City Marathon.

Now we take Mats to some of the local fun runs on occasion, and I see a lot of parents pushing their kids to run faster and longer. I don't believe in a child actually doing running workouts. They stay fit simply by playing games with the other neighborhood kids. Soccer is a great cardiovascular workout. I believe any kid who plays soccer can run a mile or two at a fun run simply by taking off the shin guards and putting on a race number.

Running on pavement is jarring to the joints and the bones, however. You have to be careful not to overdo running on pavement with your kids, because their bones and joints are incredibly fragile while they are still growing. There is not much in the way of "give" in concrete. Run in the park, on the grass or dirt, as much as possible. Use well-maintained trails—ones with few bumps and roots. Don't expect your kids to pay attention to the ground the same way you would. Look ahead and steer them away from trouble.

In my opinion, less is more when it comes to running with your children. Use good judgment and err on the side of safety and sanity. I would much rather have Mats still running when he's twenty-five than burn him out at ten.

Julie: Being a Fitness Parent I used to run up and down the coast pushing the Baby Jogger. I brought a spare diaper, sunscreen, a snack and a drink for Mats, and a water bottle for myself. It was a great way to maximize Mats's naptime. Sometimes I could run for an hour while Mats slept in the Jogger. The movement seemed to help him sleep.

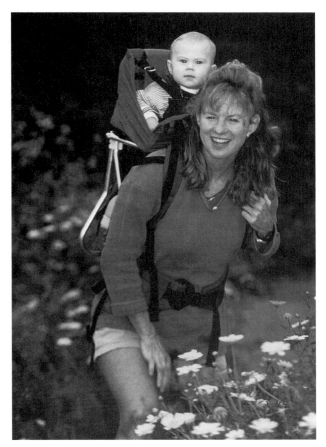

There is no reason to let becoming a mother slow you down. Mats and Julie had some great times out on the hiking trails.

Being creative with your time is goal number one as a fitness parent.

At first, we were hesitant to take the Jogger out on the trails, figuring it would be too bouncy for the baby. How wrong we were! For Mats, it was like an E-ticket ride at Disneyland. All the whoop-de-doos of the trails made it fun for him, and his laughing and shrieking made going off-road even more enjoyable for both Mark and me.

When we went exploring into the local canyons, we saw cows and sheep and hawks. We could stop and share those moments with Mats. Rather than learning about nature from a book, he was learning from firsthand experience. I look back on some of those off-road runs around our local lagoon and realize now just how special they were.

Our friends Mike and Marci Pigg had twins a

year or so ago. Marci told me that she likes to take the twins out in the Baby Jogger but, instead of running, she likes to in-line skate with the kids. I don't know how much in-line skating you have done, but it scares the heck out of me. You have a small piece of rubber on the back of one of your skates and you have to lift your toe up and drag this thing across the ground to stop. I'm not quite secure enough in my ability to stay upright to trust my safety to that small piece of rubber. So when Marci told me that she was skating with her kids, I was skeptical.

Yet Marci pointed out that she feels a lot more secure skating with the Jogger than without it. The Jogger has a hand brake on it that is a lot like the ones we have on our bikes, so Marci is actually more in control when she skates with the twins than she would be on her own.

Mark: Setting an Example Since Mats was born, he has seen Julie and me head out the door for runs almost every day. Already he asks *us* to take him for a run. You can't expect to have an active kid unless you're an active parent. You have to teach by example.

Even before his first jog, Mats was swimming. Fearless to the point of danger, he would jump into the pool in water well over his head into our arms. Now he has the skills to be water-safe, and he mimics our training, going back and forth in the pool.

These things are fun for him. They are not a workout that he is doing to get healthy. He just enjoys moving his body. And Julie and I are part of his "team" because we do more than watch him participate. We do it with him. This is what lifestyle fitness is all about.

Playing Games There are games that we like to play at home with Mats and his friends. With a bunch of kids, a park, and an hour to kill, everyone will have a blast. Start playing these games with the neighborhood kids and you will be voted mom or dad of the year. Take that to the bank.

Capture the Flag. A simple game, but a great one. You need a fairly large area to play on. Trees and boulders to hide behind are always nice.

Separate into two teams and divide the field in half. Find two T-shirts and designate them as your flags. Each team has to defend their flag and get the other team's flag over to their side of the field to win. When someone runs to your side of the field and your team tags the scoundrel, they have to go to "jail"—a tree or a rock that you designate. Remember, your goal isn't so much to dominate the five-year-olds; it's to get them and keep them running. People get released from jail if someone from the other team can tag the jail or the jailees without being touched themselves. Then everyone is free but has to go back to their side of the field before attacking the flag. The defender cannot camp out on the flag, but can be near it. It's a *great* strategy game and a *great* workout for everyone. This game can last far longer than you can. Remember to emphasize the great plays and the great runs, not just the capturing of the elusive flag. Two thumbs up from Mark and Julie.

Kick the Can. A cool dusk or nighttime game. A can or ball is placed in the center of a backyard or playground and one person is designated "It." "It" counts to 50 and then tries to find the kids who have hidden in the meantime. When "It" spots someone, she goes back to the ball or can, puts her foot on it, and announces something like, "I see Mr. Johnson in the bright orange sweater hiding behind that pole that he is three times thicker than." If you are spotted, you go to jail. If someone attacks and kicks the ball, all the prisoners go free. After a given time period, have someone else be "It" so everyone has an equal chance to be abused.

Rock-Paper-Scissors. Kids love this one. A backyard is plenty big and all ages can play. Divide into two teams. Each team huddles up and decides if they will be rock, paper, or scissors. Rock breaks scissors, scissors cut paper, and paper covers rock. Both teams approach the center line and do the rock-paper-scissors chant before putting out their sign. The side with the winning sign chases and tags anyone and everyone from the other team. Those who are tagged join the tagging team. Then both sides rehuddle and repeat. The game is over when everyone ends up on the same team.

Blob Tag/Freeze Tag. A variation on a theme. Especially with younger kids, the key is to create a variety of games. If you are planning to play for thirty minutes, you might be looking at three different ten-minute games to keep the kids' attention. Blob tag is simply your being a blob and getting bigger and bigger with each kid you catch. When they are all caught, the game is over. Freeze tag is a backyard staple. You are "It." When you tag someone, he is frozen. If someone else tags him, he becomes unfrozen. This game can last far into the next century if you let it. It's hard for Dad sometimes to remember that the point of the game is not really to freeze everyone but to keep the kids running for as long as humanly possible. If they all fall asleep at the dinner table, consider yourself an immediate inductee into the Mommy and Daddy Hall of Fame.

Organized Sports As your children get older, they'll be ready for organized sports. And a child who's already living a fit lifestyle is more likely to be successful at soccer, Little League, flag football, or gymnastics. Encourage team play—it builds character and helps a child learn how to work with others.

Go to the games, help out at the practices. The time you spend now with your child—and the children he plays with—is very important to his self-esteem and security as he enters the wider world of school and play. You'll find that it also enriches your own life. Don't push, however. Let him enjoy. Keep the pressure off. Winning isn't the point here, and you shouldn't let it become an issue.

Older children may become interested in tennis, badminton, basketball, in-line hockey, karate, or dance. Karate provides a mental discipline as well as a physical one, but you need to be sure the instructors are kid-oriented and low-key. Wrestling provides perhaps the best overall workout of any sport, although most kids (and parents) shy away from its one-on-one intensity. Many areas offer wrestling only to teenage boys.

Whatever sports your child is interested in, try to encourage her to keep playing a variety of sports and physical games. Call it cross-training for kids—it keeps her balanced both physically and emotionally.

If your kid is interested in developing her skills further than you can help her with, check into sport classes, camps, and clinics. Most larger towns offer them, although I wouldn't recommend this kind of intensive training until a child is at least ten years old. At that point, the child's natural competitiveness is likely to start surfacing, and organized sports can help direct it positively.

Kids' Sports Resource Guide

Adventure Cycling Association, (406) 721-1776

Amateur Speed Skating Union, (800) 634-4766

American Hiking Society, (301) 565-6704

American Running and Fitness Association, (800) 776-2732

American Ski Association, (800) 525-SNOW

American Youth Soccer Organization (AYSO), (800) USA-AYSO, www.soccer.org

GirlSports, (800) 643-4798. In association with the Girl Scouts, this association is for girls from five to seventeen years of age. It emphasizes overall fitness, nutrition, health, safety, leadership, and teamwork.

International In-line Skating Association, (910) 762-7004, www.1159.org

International Mountain Bike Association, (303) 545-9011

Ironkids Triathlon Series, (800) 449-4284

The Lacrosse Foundation, (410) 235-6882

Little League Baseball, www.littleleague.org

National Alliance for Youth Sports, (407) 684-1141

National Association of Governor's Councils on Physical Fitness and Sports, (317) 237-5630

National Association of Sport & Physical Education, (800) 321-0789

National Youth Coaches Association, www.nays.org

National Youth Sports Coaches Association, (800) 729-2057

President's Challenge, www.indiana.edu/-preschal

Sportsline USA, www.sportsline.com

United States Canoe Association, (513) 422-3739

United States Diving, (317) 237-6689

United States Golf Association (USGA), www.usga.org

United States Olympic Committee, (719) 632-5551

USA Cycling Federation, (719) 578-4581

USA Gymnastics Federation, (317) 237-5050

USA Hockey, (719) 599-5500

USA Track and Field, (317) 261-0500

USA Triathlon, (719) 597-9090

U.S. Rowing Association, (317) 237-5656

U.S. Sports Camps, www.us-sportscamps.com

U.S. Swimming, (719) 578-4578

U.S. Tennis Association, (914) 696-0300, www.usta.com

U.S. Water Polo, (317) 237-5599

Volleyball, www.volleyball.com

Women's Sports Foundation, www.lifetimetv.com/WoSport

XXX Sports, www.xxxsports.com

YMCA, (888) 222-9622

Youth Fitness Coalition/Project ACES, (201) 433-8993

Youth Hockey Network, www.youthhockeynetwork.com

Youth Sports Institute, (517) 353-6689

12 Body, Heart, and Spirit—How to Maintain Your Fitness Program

t's time to start tapping into the vast potential that lies waiting deep inside you. The physical part of your potential is honed by doing the physical training. Every time you go out the door for a workout, you are making deposits into the bank account of physical strength and experience. But in terms of overall health and of peak performance at races, the physical training is only part of what it takes to reach your potential.

In the fitness picture, your physical workouts could be equated to the aerobic phase of your training. They lay the groundwork for performance and results, and there is no way to get around them. Your mind and spirit, on the other hand, are the equivalent of speed work. Without speed work, your race will not reach its potential. And without the right mental at-

titude and focus, you will end up short of what you are truly capable of, whether you are talking about a race or lifetime fitness. Your mind and spirit can take you to performance realms you could only dream of on an ordinary day.

The suggestions and exercises that follow may appear very simple and obvious on the surface. But simple is better when it comes to working with thoughts and feelings. The power and impact comes from working with them over and over again. Each time you do the exercises, you will strengthen deeper parts of yourself.

It's just like going back and forth in the pool. The concept is absolutely basic—back and forth. But the result becomes profound as you do it over and over, getting in better and better shape. The same happens with mental training.

The more you do it, the better you get at accessing the power of your mind and your heart.

Your Toughest Competitor Who do you think your toughest competitor in any race is? Who do you think has the greatest chance to defeat you? Who do you think has the greatest chance of keeping you from doing your workout or losing those twenty pounds? Who will be the one person to prevent you from finishing, from achieving your goal, from feeling great about yourself, your race, your life? Who do you think can hold you back inches away from a personal victory?

It's you.

The weather is not your biggest obstacle. The demands of your boss do not ultimately pre-

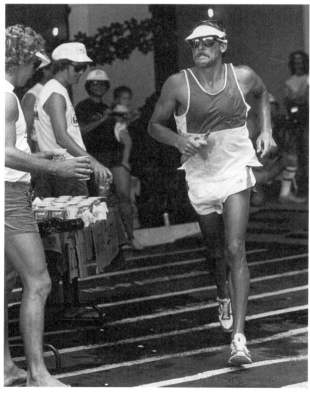

In 1984 I had a thirteen-minute lead over Dave Scott at the end of the Ironman bike ride. I thought that the race was in the bag. The guy had to gain thirty seconds per mile on me for 26.2 straight miles! You know what they say about the best-laid plans of mice and race leaders, don't you? This angry-looking guy came by me like a freight train about thirteen miles into the run. I was barely moving by then.

vent you from making it to the gym. Your family is not the guilty party that keeps you feeling half-happy, nor should they be made to feel that they are. Those are just tests along the way to help you tap into deeper and more powerful areas of yourself. Those challenges help you understand the essence of your own strength and your willingness to surrender to the task at hand. The biggest limiting factor in performance and in fulfilling your dreams, once the hard work is done, is your own attitude and ability to deal with the challenges that present themselves along the way.

Fortunately, you have the ability to change yourself. You can't change the weather, the distance of the race, or your competitor's fitness. You probably can't ignore the quotas set by your boss. You can't shove your kids in a closet while you train. But you *can* change your attitude to be positive, regardless of what is going on around you. You *can* increase your ability to face your fears. You *can* discover a way to achieve your wildest dreams.

Julie, Mark, and Mats: Fear Julie: Fear, all kinds of fear, lurks in inaction: fear of getting started, fear of failure, fear of never being able to get in shape, fear of not knowing how to make a goal happen, fear of how bad it might hurt. The only way to face fears, to transform them, is to get out there and take the first steps.

Mark: It's normal to have fear. It keeps us from doing stupid things. But it can also hold us back from having an incredible experience. My fears—about Ironman, marriage, having a child—could have kept me from giving 100 percent of what I had to give. If I had given in to my fears, even a little bit, I would not have won that race six times, I would not be with my wife, and Mats would not be here.

Mats: I'm not afraid of anything. My dad is scared if I climb high in the tree that I might fall.

Action Requires Structure Finding the right materials to build a framework for action is so important. The structure for a balanced heart, spirit, and ultimately a great race is built on a positive focus that opens the doorway to your greatest potential. Here is one way to help become conscious of how your thoughts work, and hopefully a way to track them so you can change them into something that helps instead of hinders you.

Make a mental note of the thoughts you tell yourself throughout the day. Listen to them, asking yourself the following questions: Are they positive or negative? Are they supportive of what you are trying to achieve or are they limiting you? Do they make you feel good about what you are doing, or do they somehow diminish what you have done during the day? Suppose you had to shorten a run because your work went longer than expected. Afterward, you find yourself thinking, "I wish I could have run ten miles instead of only having the time to go five." In a very subtle but powerful way, you have just told yourself that five miles wasn't enough. By telling yourself that to achieve your goal you needed ten miles, you just took the benefit of a five-mile run and made it go away. You also gave yourself an excuse for failure.

Stop yourself right there. Consciously change any negative or limiting thought you are having to a positive or supportive thought. Tell yourself—aloud if possible—"Five miles was perfect. At least I got in that much, and because I worked a little longer I now have extra time to run the next time I go out." This is a very positive way to talk to yourself about the same situation. It also signals your body that there was something good about that run, maximizing your benefit from it. It has been put in the bank.

Do this exercise for three consecutive days. Start now. For the next three days, make a real effort to change all of those negatives into positives. Find a way, no matter how ridiculous the logic seems. Change the thoughts you tell yourself regardless of whether you believe them at that exact moment or not.

If you do this, the energy and direction of your entire life will improve dramatically. It changes you by changing what you tell yourself about yourself. No one gives you more feedback throughout the day about you and your world than you do. Change that voice and the world of possibility will open up.

Mark: Giving Up Doubt I keep coming back to Brant Secunda and Huichol shamanism. The themes he talks about weave through the world of experiences that I had in sports, and the connection of the two worlds has given me the simple framework upon which the most profound experiences in my life have been built.

One of the things Brant says over and over and over is that negative thoughts hold us back from being whole people, from connecting to our world with our hearts. Anger, fear, jealousy, self-doubt all hold us back from becoming our best, from connecting to the very source of life itself. He also says to give those thoughts up because they are not really who we are anyway. Just give them up.

At the 1992 Ironman, I had to use this powerful tool. At the start of the run, I found myself trailing the best runner in the sport at that time, Christian Bustos of Chile, by about twenty seconds. I couldn't close the gap no matter how hard I tried. Finally, after several surges and many miles of running, I pulled up even with him. Unfortunately, he took one look at me and sped up.

My mind started to completely sabotage my race. I was telling myself everything negative. "Bustos is a stronger runner than I am. He is going too hard. I can't keep up with him. I can't handle this much pain. If I run this fast this early, I will surely blow up later. It's not worth it. I just can't do this anymore. He's going to win the Ironman." And so it went.

Finally, I told myself to just *shut up!* I took a mental time-out and stepped onto the sidelines inside myself. I took several deep breaths, which wasn't so easy at the pace Christian was running. Shortly after that, everything inside calmed down. I went from negative thoughts to no thoughts, and then to powerfully positive thoughts, to excitement just being in the thick of it, battling for the lead with such a fierce competitor.

A mile later my body started to loosen up slightly. Christian's pace suddenly felt easier to match, and my own stride seemed to lengthen. In the next moment, I knew it was only a matter of time before I would pull away and win my fourth title at the Ironman!

Julie: Being Consistent Having a goal of being consistent with my workouts is the best way for me to keep thoughts positive. It's fun to see how many workouts I can string together each week. It's not that I can't miss a workout here and there, it's just something fundamentally positive to focus on. If I don't work out, then I make up for it the next day. Two days off has more of a negative effect on my attitude. I can't miss three days without it affecting my thoughts—which brings it all back again to consistency keeping me positive.

Mark: Negativity More often than not, negative thoughts creep in when I lose sight of the basic things in life that I should be thankful for—my life, for starters. A bad workout looks pretty rosy compared to not being alive to work out. Yeah, that is obvious, but it can be very hard to feel when your emotions are running contrary to thoughts of thankfulness and joy.

That's one of the reasons I love to take time-outs from my life where I soak up nature. I lose my "self" when our family shares a beautiful sunset or the view of a snowcapped mountain. It makes me happy just to be alive. And that happiness is a much stronger starting point to live from than trying to build happiness and fulfillment off a base of negativity, anger, fear, or doubt. The bottom line is that it's hard to have negative thoughts when you're feeling joy.

Mats: Being Happy The most important thing is just to be happy you are alive, even if it's for a short time. Even if you only lived for one day, it's important that you lived.

It's Only an Image A negative image can hold you back—yet a negative image is an illusion. It implies something that is inherent that cannot be modified. Holding a positive self-image creates the possibility of transformation. It becomes a magnet for action. It is also a possibility for change. Everyone has some limiting or negative image. If you let that hold you back, you give it power. If you refuse to be limited by negative attitudes or perceptions, they become like

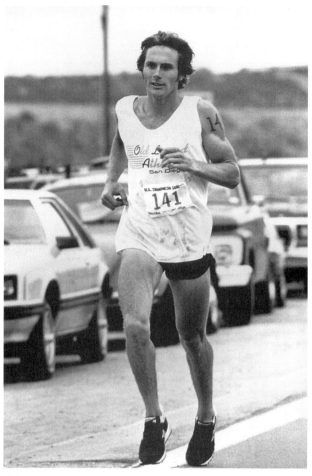

This was my breakthrough race: the first-ever United States Triathlon Series event in San Diego back in 1982. As a college swimmer, I always gave up when somebody passed me. As a runner in this race, I was passed and dropped back to fifth place. But then I gathered myself and moved back into fourth place. I really liked this new sport . . . and the new Mark Allen.

the wind that passes on by, or a light that shines onto new possibilities once reality is seen.

Directed Energy, Part One One of the best ways to keep a positive focus and have good thoughts about what we do is to direct our energy into areas that will make a positive difference. Here is a way to help do that.

Make a list of the things you feel are getting or could get in the way of achieving your goal. These could be concrete things, like job obligations. They could be more feeling-oriented things like fears you have that hold you back.

Make the list as broad and long as necessary. This is a chance for you to see what your real obstacles are—both external ones and those lurking inside you.

Now, go down the list and cross out every one of the things that you cannot change and have no control over. It will waste your precious energy to focus on these. The items remaining are the things that you can change and control. Focus on these with the full devotion of your energy.

Mark: Control What You Can

For years, I wanted the other competitors in the Ironman to have a bad race, because I couldn't see myself winning unless someone else fell apart. I also wanted the weather to be cooler, the wind to blow at my back, and the distances to be shorter.

Well, it is obvious that I don't have control over the type of race my competitors will have, nor do I control the weather. And, short of cutting the course, I was not going to decrease the distance. I was wasting my energy by focusing on those things.

In 1989, I focused my energies on getting as strong as I could be before arriving in Kona. This was something I could control. Gaining as much personal strength as possible took my focus away from hoping someone else would fall apart. I also focused on how I could stay calm and hydrated regardless of the wind or the heat on race day. The result was life-changing. I won for the first time in Hawaii.

Going Outside the Comfort Zone

We all have a zone of comfort that we generally live within. But achieving that ultimate goal might require stretching way out beyond it. First people take the action and make the changes that are comfortable, leaving the bigger problems or issues alone. Yet it's the big ones lurking outside the zone of comfort that will be waiting at the key moments of challenge.

The challenge comes at the point when you are pushed to the limit and asked—usually through the language of pain, boredom, or self-doubt—if you are willing to go beyond that comfort barrier. Doing this can be a gift. Making the stretch empowers you with an understanding about your own capabilities that you don't experience in your ordinary comfortable reality.

Directed Energy, Part Two

It's rare that the weak link is one of the easy things to change. The weakest part of you is usually the deepest, most difficult to identify. If it were easy, you would probably have fixed it long ago. Directed Energy, Part One already helped you see what things are within your control that might get in the way of accomplishing your goal. To go to the limit of your potential, the weakest link inside needs to be identified and transformed. Here is a way to do this.

Write down some of the things you think will get in the way of living your ultimate dream. Try to think of both physical and psychological limitations you feel you have.

Take the one thing from this list that you feel could have the biggest negative impact on accomplishing your goal, and ask yourself: "If I change this one thing, can I see myself accomplishing my ultimate goal?" If you still can't see yourself achieving the goal, even with this point changed, delve deeper until you come up with something even more basic that could be the key thing holding you back. Keep doing this until you discover the most elemental fear, block, or limiting component to reaching your goal.

Now it's time to go forward, adjusting and changing that key part of yourself or your life that could hold you back from your dream, and then finally realizing that dream.

Julie: A Different Perspective

I look at ways I can improve rather than what is holding me back. I am so happy to have this lifestyle, I don't dwell on the negatives. Fundamentally I know an active lifestyle is what works for me. From there everything else falls into place.

Mark: Logic and Emotion

Prior to 1989, I tried to make a logical analysis of what I

needed to change to win the Ironman. I spent much of my energy trying to change diet, training, and equipment and, by the beginning of 1989, I was on a great training program. I was eating very healthily and my equipment was state of the art. Yet I knew it still wasn't enough to win the Ironman. Although each of these were essential parts of the equation, they were also within my comfort zone of change, and none of them were my weakest link. What could it be that needed to be changed or transformed?

Then it came to me. The biggest limiting factor to my success in Kona was that I was totally and completely intimidated by everything about the Ironman. The distance intimidated me. The conditions intimidated me. I was intimidated by my competitors. In short, I was afraid of that race.

So I changed my focus away from trying to change the things that were easy and focused on changing whatever I needed to about myself to enable me to go over to Hawaii and deal with the conditions, the island, and my competitors. I changed the key problem—my own attitude.

That year's race was still hot, windy, and long. My toughest competitor raced at my side virtually the entire race. And I still felt intimidated. The significant difference was that I was able to stand fearless in the face of that insecurity. I was able to kick race-sabotaging doubt back out the minute it entered my thoughts. And I had the performance of my life, winning against my toughest competitor on his best day ever.

Julie: Getting Older As I get older, I have to remind myself that some of my past times are not going to be met again. So I don't let past standards hold me back from the positive experiences I can have right now. The reality of being a master (over forty) competitor is that I have new incentives. The parameters keep changing. I may not be a world-class runner, but I can be the best I can be right now. I cannot change the fact that I am getting older. I can affect the quality of my life.

Creating an Essential Balance There is the *ideal* of how you would like to progress along the path to your goal. There is also a *reality* of what it is going to take to make this ideal happen. *Balance* happens when the ideal of your life, of your goal, is matched with your willingness to accept the work and mindset necessary to accomplish that goal or ideal. The great marathon runner Juma Ikanga said, "The will to win means nothing without the will to prepare." When the ideal and the reality meet, incredible things happen. Here is something that can help accomplish that balance.

Write down a statement of your ideal fitness goal or race outcome. Next, sit quietly by yourself, close your eyes, and ask yourself this very simple question: "What will it take to achieve that goal?"

Now ask, "Are the things it will take to achieve this goal the same things that I am doing right now?" You will probably find some things that are helping to drive you in the direction of achieving the goal and some things that need to be changed if you are going to achieve it.

Follow this up by imagining yourself changing the things you just identified that are inconsistent with realizing your dream. Now, go back and see if that will be enough to make the ideal come true. If it seems like it's enough, congratulations. Go out there, change them, and keep going.

If it still seems that there is a difference between your ideal and the reality of your life, keep working with these changes in your mind until you get as close as you can to seeing yourself at that moment of fulfillment. If you just cannot seem to clear the road on your internal landscape to get the reality of your life to match your ideal, it's time for a reality check. You may have to change the ideal. Restructure your ideal statement to match the reality of your life. From there, go out and conquer!

Mark: Connecting the Dream with Reality Before the 1989 Ironman, I had gone over to Kona with the ideal statement, "I want to win the Ironman." It was very simple, very clear. But the reality wasn't matching up with my ideal. I was coming away with disasters

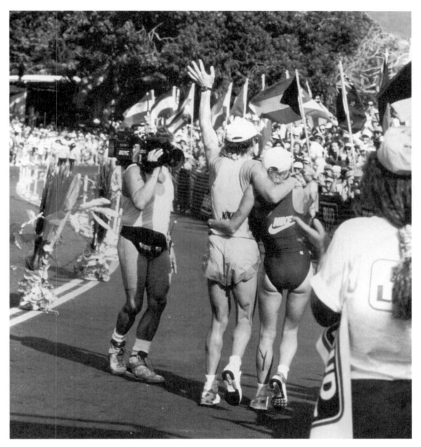

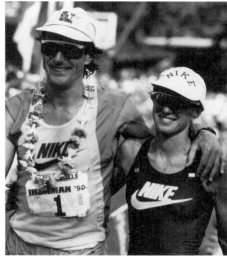

You know what feels great? Having a goal, sharing that goal with a loved one, and then reaching it. 1990 was the second year in a row that Julie and I made a plan for the year, stuck with it, and came away with an Ironman victory. It was never just Mark Allen winning the Ironman: It was Julie, Mats, my family and friends. The same goes for you and your fitness. To be successful you need to make it a team effort.

every time I started. Flat tires, walking on the marathon, even internal bleeding one year were keeping me from living that ideal dream to win.

I had to ask myself *why?* Why could I win everywhere else in the world but not at the Ironman? I looked more closely at my ideal statement. There was something I was subconsciously and silently adding on to the end of my ideal statement. My full ideal statement was, "I want to win the Ironman, but only if I can do it and stay in my comfort zone." The reality was that my comfort zone was far below what it would take to win.

To get the ideal and the reality of that goal to match, I had to restructure my ideal statement. I changed it to say, "I want to win the Ironman *and* I am willing to do whatever it takes on all levels to do it." Now, my ideal and the reality of the situation were in balance.

The effect was profound on my entire approach. I trained for six weeks in New Zealand with Julie in what became a daily discovery of new levels in distance and speed. My focus changed from trying to do what it would take to win to training at a level that would take me to a win *plus* about another 20 percent. Something always goes wrong at the Ironman, and if you only trained to cross the finish line just ahead of your competitor, there is no room for error—which is a huge error in training strategy.

The race that year became known as Iron War. I pulled away from six-time champion Dave Scott in the last mile to win my first Ironman title. The roughly 20 percent increase in my strategic training translated into a winning margin of less than a minute in a race that took over eight hours to complete.

Julie: Balance Balance is really about making your life work—your *whole* life. It's recognizing all that I am: a woman, a wife, a mother, and an athlete. Each day I juggle all of these roles around, giving each one the time and energy that is needed.

One of my faults is that I overprogram. I tend to keep my days too full and I get overwhelmed with how to keep everything in order. Every once in a while I have a meltdown, which forces me to get back to simplicity. If we don't have the time to stop long enough to watch sunset as a family, I know it's time to reassess and make some changes.

Entering the Zone of Discovery You may be familiar with Discovery by other names or definitions. Some call it a meditative state. Others would say it is a state where directed conscious intellectual thought is replaced with action that simply seems to happen through intuition. It is the same as being "in the zone," that state where you somehow block out all the distractions that could keep you from achieving your ultimate goal. Instead of seeing the potential for failure, your focus becomes whole and complete on seeing your goal happening. Doubts and fears take a backseat to confidence, understanding, potential, and the possibility that something magic can happen beyond your normal guidelines of reality.

This is the state of *Discovery*. In shamanism, it is referred to as the space between two thoughts where your intuition takes over, where you are connected to the memory of cre-

ation itself. It's a quiet alertness where answers come and life is created in just about any way you can imagine it. It is total absorption in making the unimaginable and impossible happen. It is the ability to keep calm under pressure. It is the ability to let fears fall by the wayside because no room exists for them in your focus and attention. In Discovery, you are too busy functioning at your highest level to have enough energy left over to contemplate failure. You stop being a part of the reality that something can go wrong. You forget about you, and transform yourself into the action of achieving your goal, of creating possibility and positive reality moment by moment.

Undoubtedly, you have experienced this state before, even though you may not have understood what was going on. Try to recall situations where things were flowing along without any need to put conscious thought into making them happen. You may have felt this during a workout, for example, where everything was firing and your body was running smoothly. You felt almost like an observer along for the ride, instead of the conductor having to direct the whole experience. This is the state of Discovery. This is what you will want to remember when you are challenged during training, racing, or life. Getting into this state is some-

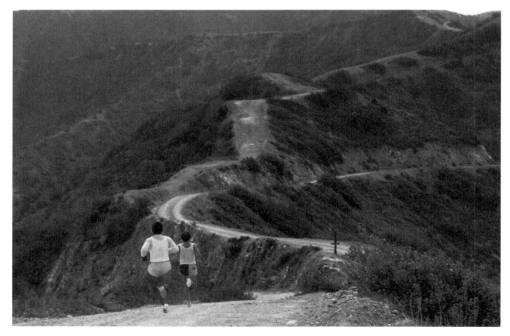

This is one of my favorite photos. There is nothing better than combining fitness with a little adventure. Find an out-of-the-way place to hike, run, mountain bike, or kayak. Then bring some training buddies and create your own personal adventure. This particular photo was taken on Catalina Island off the coast of Los Angeles.

thing you can be practicing every day. Here is an example of how to do it.

The next time you are in a situation that is uncomfortable or challenging, watch for panic, anger, frustration, or any physical tightening. This is *not* the state of Discovery. These are the average person's responses to challenge. Brainwave activity increases; body functions start to lean toward handling stress and getting ready for fight or flight.

Once you see these things happening, stop yourself. Stop whatever mental chatter is happening. Stop panicking. Take a mental step outside of the situation and set yourself on the sidelines for a moment. Take several deep, slow breaths and calm your mind so that it feels as though your brain activity is even less than normal daily levels. You should start to feel similar to when you are relaxing in bed just before sleep. This is the state of Discovery. This state is what exceptional athletes enter into when confronted with competition stress and race chaos.

Now ask yourself what needs to be done to move beyond the challenge at hand and keep you on track to achieving your ultimate goal. The answer that comes may surprise you, but it will be the correct one—because it came to you in a state of calm, a state of Discovery, from the space between two thoughts. With this calm and the answer, reenter the arena.

Practice this during workouts when it gets tough. Try it out when your boss begins to panic and blames a bad situation on you. Use this tool when it seems like neither you nor your mate can come up with any logical solution to lack of workout time and you are both grumpy. Make mental notes of what it feels like to be in this state, where you can be calm even though chaos may be happening around you. The more you experience this state, the easier it will be to enter it. Ultimately, you will be able to access this state naturally whenever challenging moments arise.

Julie: A Quiet Mind It doesn't happen that often, but when it does, it's usually on a long run. I've exhausted all those conversations going on in my head, and physically I'm near my limit. My body is demanding all my attention, so my mind is forced to be quiet so as not to distract from the task at hand.

Some people call this *the zone*. It's not about concentration. It happens when I am quiet, when I stop trying with my mind. These flashes that happen in a workout can be short, but they are priceless. You're completely in the moment and standing back in awe as you watch yourself run the last mile faster than the first. It's the running equivalent of a spiritual experience.

Mark: Discovery Moments of quiet can happen when you are exercising. At these times, you find new strengths that were not available before. Such discoveries happen when you have the courage to go into a zone that holds your fear, ego, and doubt—somewhere on the other side of your comfort zone.

The Tools You now have many tools that can be used to intensify your physical potential. Here is a quick refresher of what they are.

• Build a structure for incredible potential from positive thoughts.

• Maximize the use of your energy by focusing on the things you can control.

• Further maximize your energy by identifying the weakest link in your game plan that is holding you back, whether it is physical, mental, or spiritual.

• Create an essential balance between the reality of what it will take to accomplish your ideal goal with what you are willing to do to make it happen.

• Enter the magical state of Discovery and use your intuition by quieting your mind, being alert, and finding that space between two thoughts.

Resources

Retreats and Fitness Seminars

Dance of the Deer Foundation Center for Shamanic Studies

The Foundation sponsors seminars, pilgrimages, and ongoing study groups throughout the world, particularly in the United States and Europe. These programs are often held at beautiful and sacred places of power. They emphasize the importance of ceremony for personal well-being and the continued survival of the environment.

Sport and Spirit is one program offered, combining the transformational power of shamanism with the essential tools necessary to achieve optimal physical health.
P.O. Box 699
Soquel, California 95073
(831) 475-9560
www.shamanism.com

Associations for Almost Every Sport

Adventure Travel
National Parks and Conservation Association
1776 Massachusetts Ave. N.W. #200
Washington, DC 20036
(202) 223-6722

Outdoor Recreation Coalition of America (ORCA)
P.O. Box 1319
Boulder, CO 80306
(303) 444-3353
e-mail info@orca.org.
www.orca.org

Aerobics and Fitness

Aerobics and Fitness Association of America (AFAA)

Aerobics instructor and personal trainer certification.
15250 Ventura Blvd. #200
Sherman Oaks, CA 91403
(800) 445-5950 ext. 600
e-mail afaa@pop3.com
www.afaa.com

American Aerobic Association International (AAAI)

Aerobics instructor and personal trainer certification.
P.O. Box 663
New Hope, PA 18938
(609) 397-2139, www.aaai-ismafitness.com

American College of Sports Medicine

Health/fitness instructor training, rehabilitation training.
P.O. Box 1440
Indianapolis, IN 46206-1440
(317) 637-9200, www.acsm.org

American Council on Exercise (ACE)

Aerobics instructor and personal trainer certification.
P.O. Box 910449
San Diego, CA 92191-0449
(800) 825-3636
e-mail acefitness@acefitness.org
www.acefitness.org

International Dance-Exercise Association (IDEA)

Aerobics conventions, trade shows; offers insurance, newsletters.
6190 Cornerstone Ct. East #204
San Diego, CA 92121
(800) 999-4332
www.ideafit.com

Jump Start, Inc.

Aerobics instructor training.
(847) 742-9964

The Pilates Studio

Training and certification in the Pilates method of exercising.
2121 Broadway #201
New York, NY 10023
(800) 4-PILATES

Baseball

U.S.A. Baseball

National governing body for amateur baseball.
3400 E. Camino Campestre
Tucson, AZ 85716
(520) 327-9700
www.usabaseball.com

Basketball

USA Basketball
5465 Mark Dabling Blvd.
Colorado Springs, CO 80918-3842
(719) 590-4800
www.usabasketball.com

Bike Outfitters

Backroads

National and international bicycle vacations, also cross-country skiing, walking, running.
(800) GO-ACTIVE

Bicycle Adventures

Bike trips in Oregon, Washington, California, Hawaii, and British Columbia.
(800) 443-6060

CBT Bike Tours

European bike tours offered for all levels, hiking and mountain biking.
415 W. Fullerton, #1003
Chicago, IL 60614
(773) 404-1710

Euro-Bike Tours

Thematic tours through Europe, offered to three levels of cyclists and walkers.
Box 990
DeKalb, IL 60115
(815) 758-8851

Imagine Tours

Cycling adventures.
P.O. Box 475
Davis, CA 95617
(888) 592-BIKE

Michigan Bicycle Touring

Biking, canoeing, kayaking, hiking.
3512 Red School
Kingsley, MI 49649
(616) 263-5885

Northwest Passage

Regional, national, and international cycling programs.

(800) RECREATE

Pow Wow Bicycle Tours

Midwestern bike tours.

(414) 671-4560

Timberline Bicycle Tours

Western U.S., Alaska, and Canadian bicycle tours.

7975 E. Howard, #J

Denver, CO 80237

(800) 417-2453

Boardsailing

U.S. Windsurfing Association

P.O. Box 978

Hood River, OR 97031

(541) 386-8708

e-mail uswa@aol.com

www.uswindsurfing.gorge.net

Bodybuilding

International Federation of Bodybuilders

2875 Bates Rd.

Montreal, Quebec, H3S 1B7 Canada

(514) 731-3783, www.ifb.com

Cycling

Adventure Cycling Association

P.O. Box 8308-P

Missoula, MT 59807

(406) 721-1776

e-mail Acabike@aol.com

www.adv-cycling.org

The Bicycle Council

P.O. Box 407

Lindon Station, WI 53944

(888) 228-8078

Bicycle Federation of America

1506 21st St. #200 NW

Washington, D.C. 20036

(202) 463-6622

Bikes Belong Steering Committee

1100 17th St. NW, 10th Floor

Washington, DC 20006

(202) 331-9696

IMBA

P.O. Box 7578

Boulder, CO 80306

(303) 545-9011

International Human-Powered Vehicle Association

Organization for recumbents, etc.

260 S. Channing #1

Elgin, IL 60120

(847) 742-5818 (contact Len Brunkalla)

International Mountain Biking Association

Nonprofit group that promotes mountain biking.

P.O. Box 7578

Boulder, CO 80306

(303) 545-9011

e-mail Imba@aol.com

www.imba.com

League of American Bicyclists

National membership organization.

1612 K Street NW, Ste. 401

Washington, D.C., 20006

(202) 822-1333, www.bikeleague.org

National Bicycle Dealers Association (NBDA)

2240 University Dr. #130

Newport Beach, CA 92660

(949) 722-6909

National Off-Road Bicycle Association (NORBA)

National governing body for mountain biking.

USA Cycling: Attn. NORBA

One Olympic Plaza

Colorado Springs, CO 80909

(719) 578-4581, www.usacycling.org

Police Mountain Bike Association

Part of the League of American Bicyclists.

1612 K St. NW, #401

Washington, D.C., 20036

(202) 822-1333

Rails to Trails Conservancy

Organized to promote conversion of abandoned rail corridors to trails for public use.

1100 17th St. NW, 10th Floor

Washington, D.C. 20036

(202) 331-9696, www.railtrails.org

Ultra Marathon Cycling Association

Promotes long-distance cycling and racing.

P.O. Box 53

Canyon, TX 79105

(805) 499-3210

United States Cycling Federation
Governing body for amateur cycling.
One Olympic Plaza,
Colorado Springs, CO 80909-5775
(719) 578-4581

United States Professional Cycling Federation
Governing body for professional cycling.
One Olympic Plaza
Colorado Springs, CO 80909
(719) 578-4581

Fencing
United States Fencing Association
One Olympic Plaza
Colorado Springs, CO 80809-5774
(719) 578-4511

Footbag/Hackey-Sack
World Footbag Association
Players Association.
P.O. Box 775208
Steamboat Springs, CO 80477
(970) 870-9898
www.worldfootbag.com

Golf
United States Golf Association
Governing body for amateur golfers.
P.O. Box 708
Liberty Corner Rd.
Far Hills, NJ 07931
(908) 234-2300
www.usga.org

Hiking
American Hiking Society
Advocacy group for the use and development of trails.
1422 Fenwick
Silver Springs, MD 20910
(301) 565-6704

Hot Air Balloons
Balloon Federation of America
112 E. Salem
P.O. Box 400
Indianola, IA 50125
(515) 961-8809
www.bfa.ycg.org

Ice Hockey
USA Hockey
National governing body for ice hockey.
1775 Bob Johnson Dr.
Colorado Springs, CO 80906
(719) 576-8724
e-mail: usah@usahockey.org

Ice Skating
The Ice Skating Institute of America (ISIA)
17120 N. Dallas Pkwy. #140
Dallas, TX 75248
(972) 735-8800
www.skateisi.com

In-line Skating
International In-Line Skating Association (IISA)
201 N. Front St., #306
Wilmington, NC 28401
(910) 762-7004
www.iisa.org

IISA Instructor Certification Program (ICP)
201 N. Front St., #306,
Wilmington, NC 28401
(910) 762-7004

USA Rollerskating
National governing body for amateur skating.
4730 South St.
P.O. Box 6579
Lincoln, NE 68506
(402) 483-7551
www.usacrs.com

Luge
Canada Olympic Park
Calgary, Canada
(403) 247-5452

Marquette Negaunee Luge Association
  Marquette, MI
  (906) 475-5843
Muskegon Luge Club
  North Muskegon, MI
  (616) 744-9629
Olympic Regional Development Authority
  Lake Placid, NY
  (518) 523-2071
U.S. Luge Association
  (518) 523-2071
Utah Winter Sports Park Bob/Luge Track
  Park City, UT
  (435) 658-4200

Olympics

United States Olympic Committee
  One Olympic Plaza
  Colorado Springs, CO 80909
  (719) 632-5551

Paddle Sports

American Canoe Association
  National organization that sanctions competitive canoe races and clubs and certifies canoe instructors.
  7432 Alban Station Blvd. #B232
  Springfield, VA 22150
  (703) 451-0141
  www.aca-paddler.org
The Professional Paddle Sports
  U.S. 27 & Hornbeck Rd.
  P.O. Box 248
  Butler, KY 41006
  (606) 472-2205
  www.propaddle.com
U.S. Canoe and Kayak Team
  2,200 members, must be a member to compete in races.
  421 Old Military Rd.
  Lake Placid, NY 12946
  (518) 523-1855
U.S. Rowing Association
  National governing body for the sport of rowing.
  201 S. Capitol Ave. #400
  Indianapolis, IN 46225
  (317) 237-5656
  www.usrowing.org

Running/Track and Field

American Running and Fitness Association
  Not-for-profit organization to educate runners and other fitness enthusiasts.
  4405 E/W Highway #405
  Bethesda, MD 20814
  (800) 776-2732
  www.arfa.org
Association of Road Racing Athletes
  Coordinates a series of prize money events for professional distance runners.
  P.O. Box 21021
  Spokane, WA 99201
Road Runner Clubs of America (RRCA)
  National association of running clubs.
  219 W. Elm
  Winona, IL 61377
  (815) 853-4547 (contact Chris Christian)
USA Track and Field
  National governing body for road racing, cross country, track and field, and race-walking events.
  P.O. Box 120
  Indianapolis, IN 46206
  (317) 261-0500

Sailing

U.S. Sailing Association
  National governing body for sailing.
  P.O. Box 1260
  Portsmouth, RI 02871
  (401) 683-0800
  www.ussailing.org

Scuba

Professional Association of Diving Instructors (PADI)
  Divers certification.
  30151 Tomas St.
  Rancho Santa Margarita, CA 92688
  (800) 729-7234
  www.padi.com
Scuba Schools International (SSI)
  Scuba certification.
  2619 Canton Ct.
  Fort Collins, CO 80525
  (970) 482-0883
  www.ssi.com

YMCA National Scuba Program

Diver certification.

5825-2A Live Oak Pkwy.

Norcross, GA 30093

(770) 662-5172

www.ymcascuba.org

Skiing

American Blind Skiing Foundation

227 E. North Ave.

Elmhurst, IL 60127

(630) 833-5892

NASTAR

c/o World Wide Ski Corporation

402-D AABC

Aspen, CO 81611

(970) 925-7864

Over the Hill Gang

Ski organization, trips, and discounts for those fifty and up.

(719) 389-0022

Professional Ski Instructors of America

133 S. Van Gordon St. #101

Lakewood, CO 80228

(303) 987-9390

70+ Ski Club

1633 Albany St.

Schenectady, NY 12304

(518) 346-5505 (contact Richard Lambert)

SnowSports Industries America (SIA)

(703) 556-9020

Winter sports hotline (703) 506-4232

U.S. Skiing

P.O. Box 100

Park City, UT 84060

(435) 649-9090

Skydiving

United States Parachute Association

National governing body.

1440 Duke St.

Alexandria, VA 22314

www.uspa.org

Soccer

U.S. Soccer Federation

Governing body for soccer.

1801-1811 S. Prairie Ave.

Chicago, IL 60616

(312) 808-1300

Speed Skating

Amateur Speedskating Union (ASU)

National governing body.

(630) 790-3230 (contact Shirley Yates)

Swimming

Aquatic Exercise Association

Resource center for aquatic fitness (vertical exercise in the pool).

P.O. Box 1609

Nokomis, FL 34274

(941) 486-8600

www.aeawave.com

Northern/Central California Masters

Novato, CA (415) 892-0771

San Diego/Imperial Masters Swimming

(619) 275-1292

Southern California Masters

Santa Monica, CA (310) 451-6666

United States Lifesaving Association

Administrative headquarters.

P.O. Box 366

Huntington Beach, CA 92648

(714) 968-9360

U.S. Swimming

One Olympic Plaza

Colorado Springs, CO 80809

(719) 578-4578

Triathlon

Ironman Mainland Office

World Triathlon Corp.

P.O. Box 1608

Tarpon Springs, FL 34688

(813) 942-4767

USA Triathlon Federation

3595 E. Fountain Blvd. #F-1

Colorado Springs, CO 80910

(727) 597-9090

Membership services (800) 874-1872

Ultimate Frisbee

Ultimate Players Association
Governing body for Ultimate Frisbee.
3595 E. Fountain Blvd. #J-2
Colorado Springs, CO 80910
(800) 872-4384
www.upa.org

Volleyball

USA Volleyball Association
Governing body for amateur hardcourt volleyball.
3595 E. Fountain Blvd. #I-2
Colorado Springs, CO 80910
(719) 637-8300

Walking

American Walking Association
Education and networking.
P.O. Box 4
Paonia, CO 81428
(303) 447-0156

USA Track and Field
Sanctioning body for race-walking.
P.O. Box 120
Indianapolis, IN 46206
(317) 261-0500

Weightlifting

U.S.A. Weightlifting Federation
National governing body.
One Olympic Plaza
Colorado Springs, CO 80909-5764
(719) 578-4508

Manufacturers

Bicycle Trailers

Bobike Cycling Carriers
(800) 586-3332
Kool-Stop Trailer
(800) 586-3332

Jogging Strollers

Kool-Stop International, Inc.
P.O. Box 3480
La Habra, CA 90632
(800) 586-3332
Kool Stride Jogging Strollers
(714) 738-4971

Shoe Manufacturers

Information numbers to find retailers near you:
Adidas: (800) 448-1796
Asics: (800) 678-9435
Avia: (888) 855-AVIA
Brooks: (800) 2-BROOKS
Etonic: (800) 334-0008
New Balance: (800) 253-SHOE
Nike: (800) 352-NIKE
Reebok: (800) 648-5550
Saucony: (800) 365-4933

Hot Sports Links

www.acefitness.org
American Council on Exercise. Become certified, membership info, read fit facts, news releases, find a certified professional.

www.activeusa.com
Nationwide source for thousands of participatory sports events.

www.adventuresports.com

Outdoor events/festivals, products, publications, organizations info, calendars, outdoor resources, trail talk, women's sports, etc.

www.fitnesszone.com

Shop here for bikes, free weights, aerobic supplies, etc. Obtain free fitness profiles, on-line fitness articles, gym locator (locate any gym in the United States). Read fitness forums, classifieds, fitness library.

www.halhigdon.com

Marathon training guides, tips, insights into marathons, training to improve your 5K and 10K races.

www.menshealth.com

Men's Health archives, read recent issues, send flowers, ask the Sex Doctor, ask *Men's Health*, surveys, games, quizzes, ask Jimmy the Bartender, Men's Health Gear, Gym Finder, other links.

www.netmarket.com

On-line sporting good superstore—order shoes, equipment, clothing accessories.

www.runnersworld.com

Training tips, recent issue articles, nutrition tips, travel, statistics, shoes, awards, forums, injury prevention tips, and descriptions.

www.serioussports.com

Comprehensive guide to the best outdoor outfitters, schools, guides, travel, adventure clubs, programs, water, air, land sports, bookstore; join an outdoor sporting goods auction—"Live to Play."

www.sports-medicine.com

Preventing injuries, search for your injury, ask Dr. Zeman, exercise, accidents and legal medicine, career links in sports medicine.

Marathons

Winter

Almost Heaven Marathon

Charleston, WV

(304) 744-6502

Andrew Jackson Marathon and 5K

USATF certified, in 1998 131 participants.

Jackson, TN

(901) 668-1708

e-mail reginaas@earthlink.net

Atlanta Marathon

Atlanta, GA

(404) 231-9065

www.atlantatrackclub.org

Big Sur Trail Marathon

Andrew Molera State Park, CA

(415) 868-1829

www.envirosports.com

Blue Angel Marathon and 5K

USATF certified, in 1998 1,100 participants.

Pensacola, FL

(850) 452-4391

www.mwr-pcola.navy.mil/current/golf-run/b_a_m_99.htm

California International Marathon

USATF certified, in 1998 3,500 participants.

Sacramento, CA

(916) 983-4622

www.runcim.org

Cape Cod Times Marathon

Hyannis, MA

(508) 775-8877

Carolina Marathon and 10K

USATF certified, in 1998 1,500 participants.

Columbia, SC

(803) 929-1996

e-mail cma@cyberstate.infi.net

www.carolinamarathon.org

Cascading Cataracts Trail Marathon

Stinson Beach, CA

(415) 868-1829

www.envirosports.com

Chickamauga Battlefield Marathon

Chickamauga, GA

(423) 875-3642

www.mindspring.com/~runchattanooga

Christmas Marathon
USATF certified.
Olympia, WA
(360) 236-7852

Columbus Marathon
USATF certified, in 1998 4,200 participants.
Columbus, OH
(614) 433-0395
e-mail racedir@aol.com
www.columbusmarathon.com

Cowtown Marathon
Fort Worth, TX
(817) 735-2033
www.cowtownmarathon.org

Cross Corral Classic Marathon
Midland, TX
(915) 689-7706

Dallas White Rock Marathon
Dallas, TX
(214) 528-2962
www.whiterock-marathon.com

Death Valley Borax Trail Marathon
Death Valley, CA
(415) 868-1829
www.envirosports.com

Death Valley Trail Marathon
Death Valley, CA
(415) 868-1829
www.envirosports.com

Delaware Marathon
USATF certified, in 1998 350 participants.
Middletown, DE
(302) 654-6400
waynek@bellatlantic.net

Desert Classic Marathon
Scottsdale, AZ
(602) 954-8341
www.arizonaroadracers.com/dclassicmar.htm

Escape from Marin Trail Marathon
Sausalito, CA
(415) 868-1829
www.envirosports.com

Gobbler Grind Marathon
Overland Park, KS
(913) 469-4090

Hampden-Sydney Marathon
Hampden-Sydney, VA
(804) 223-6178
ceres.hsc.edu/HSmarathon.html

Harrisburg Marathon
Harrisburg, PA
(717) 761-5178

Honolulu Marathon
USATF certified.
Oahu, HI
(808) 734-7200
e-mail info@honolulumarathon.org
www.honolulumarathon.org

Hudson Mohawk Marathon
Albany, NY
(518) 435-4500

Jacksonville Marathon
Jacksonville, FL
(904) 739-1917
www.1stplacesports.com

Kentucky Marathon
Louisville, KY
(502) 228-1133

Kiawah Island Marathon
USATF certified.
Kiawah Island, SC
(843) 768-6001

Las Vegas International Marathon, Half-Marathon and 5K
USATF certified, in 1998 900 participants.
Las Vegas, NV
(702) 876-3870
e-mail lvmarathon@aol.com
www.lvmarathon.com

Leprechaun Marathon
Vandalia, OH
(937) 898-7015

Lost Soles Marathon
Talent, OR
(541) 535-4854

Marathon Six Pack
Six marathons in six days.
Vandalia, OH
(937) 898-7015 (contact Denny Fryman)

Memphis Marathon
Memphis, TN
(800) 893-7223
www.runmemphis.com

Methodist Health Care Houston Marathon and 5K
Houston, TX
(713) 957-3453
www.houstonmarathon.com

Mid-Winter Marathon
Huber Heights, OH
(937) 898-7015

Mississippi Coast Marathon
Ocean Springs, MS
(228) 875-6855

Mississippi Marathon
Clinton, MS
(601) 856-9884

Morgan Hill Marathon
Morgan Hill, CA
(408) 997-3581
e-mail calsports@earthlink.com

Motorola Austin Marathon
Austin, TX
(512) 505-8304
www.motorolamarathon.com

New York City Marathon
USATF certified.
New York, NY
(212) 423-2249
www.nyrrc.org

Nokia Sugar Bowl Mardi Gras Marathon, Half Marathon and 5K
New Orleans, LA
(504) 482-6682

Northern Central Trail Marathon
Sparks, MD
(410) 668-8653

Ocala Marathon
Ocala, FL
(352) 732-4833

Ocean State Marathon
USATF certified.
Narragansett, RI
(401) 885-4499
www.osm26.com

Official All Star Cafe Myrtle Beach Marathon
5-person relay, USATF certified, in 1998 2,500 participants.
Myrtle Beach, SC
(843) 293-RACE
www.coastal.edu/mbmarathon

Olympiad Memorial Marathon
St. Louis, MO
(314) 434-9577

Philadelphia Marathon
Philadelphia, PA
(215) 685-0054
www.philadelphiamarathon.com

Richmond Marathon
Richmond, VA
(804) 673-7223
www.rrc.org

San Antonio Marathon
USATF certified, 1998 1,200 participants.
San Antonio, TX
(210) 648-9383
www.samarathon.org

San Diego Marathon, Half-Marathon, 5K and Bike Tour
Carlsbad, CA
(619) 792-2900 (contact In Motion)

Santa Clarita Marathon
USATF certified.
Santa Clarita, CA
(888) 823-3455
scrunners.org/marathon

Seattle Marathon
USATF certified.
Seattle, WA
(206) 729-3660

Smoky Mountain Marathon and 5K
In 1998 500 participants.
Townsend, TN
(423) 588-7465
www.ktc.org

Space Coast Marathon
Melbourne, FL
(407) 784-3050

Stinson Beach Trail Marathon
Mt. Tamalpais State Park & Muir Woods National Park, CA
(415) 868-1829
www.envirosports.com

Tucson Marathon, Half Marathon and Relay
Tucson, AZ
(520) 320-0667

Tybee Marathon
Tybee Island, GA
(912) 921-4786 (day) or 232-0070 (evening)

Vulcan Marathon
USATF certified.
Birmingham, AL
(800) 266-5426
www.run42k.com

Washington's Birthday Marathon and Relay
USATF certified, in 1998 300 participants.
Greenbelt, MD
(703) 241-0395,
patriot.net/~dcrrc/gwm.html

Western Hemisphere Marathon
Culver City, CA
(310) 253-6668

WZYP Rocket City Marathon
USATF certified, in 1998 1,000 participants.
Huntsville, AL
(256) 828-6207
www.huntsvilletrackclub.org

Spring

Andy Payne Marathon
Oklahoma City, OK
(405) 236-2800
e-mail unity@unityinc.org

Army Medcom Marathon and Relays
Fort Sam Houston, TX
(210) 221-2523

Athens Marathon
USATF certified.
Athens, Ohio
(740) 594-3825
www.athensohio.com

Avenue of the Giants Marathon and 10K
Send self-addressed stamped envelope for info to:
281 Hidden Valley Rd.
Bayside, CA 95524
www.humboldt1.com/~avenue

BAA Boston Marathon
USATF certified, in 1998 11,500 participants.
Hopkinton, MA to Boston
(508) 435-6905
e-mail mile27@star.net,
www.bostonmarathon.org

B&A Trail Marathon
USATF certified, in 1998 600 participants.
Severna Park, MD
(410) 987-0674
e-mail tabslab@aol.com

Bayshore Marathon
Traverse City, MI
(616) 941-8118
users.northlink.net/tctc (contact Dave Taylor)

Big Basin Redwoods Trail Marathon
Santa Cruz, CA
(415) 868-1829
www.envirosports.com

Big Sur Marathon
USATF certified.
Carmel, CA
(408) 625-6226
e-mail info@bsim.org
www.bsim.org

Buffalo Marathon
Buffalo, NY
www.doitsports.com/buffalo

Camp Lejeune Marathon
Camp Lejeune, NC
(910) 451-1799

Cannon Long Island Marathon
USATF certified, in 1998 8,000 participants.
East Meadow, NY
(516) 572-0251

Capital City Marathon
Olympia, WA
(360) 786-1786
www.ontherun.com

Catalina Marathon
Two Harbors, CA
(714) 978-1528
www.pacificllc.com

Charlotte Observer Marathon
Charlotte, NC
(704) 358-5425
www.charlotte.com/marathon

City of Pittsburgh Marathon
Pittsburgh, PA
(412) 647-7866
www.upmc.edu/pghmarathon

Coeur d'Alene Marathon
Coeur d'Alene, ID
(208) 665-9393

CVS Cleveland Marathon and 10K
USATF certified.
Cleveland, OH
(800) 467-3826
www.cvs.com/investors/marathon/index.html

Dallas Trails Marathon
Dallas, TX
(214) 324-4304

Ellerbe Springs Marathon
Ellerbe Springs, NC
(910) 895-2626

Flora London Marathon
London, Great Britain
(44) 161 703 8547

Flying Pig Marathon
USATF certified.
Cincinnati, OH
(513) 721-7447
www.cincymarathon.org

Forest City Marathon
London, Ontario, Canada
(519) 685-8675

14th Annual MCRD Marathon Relay
5 legs of 5.3 miles each.
San Diego, CA
(619) 524-6058

Glass City Marathon
USATF certified, in 1998 650 participants.
Toledo, OH
(419) 475-0731 (contact Tom Falvey)

Golden Gate Headlands Marathon
Trials in Golden Gate National Recreation Area.
Sausalito, CA
(415) 868-1829 (contact EnviroSports)

Great Potato Marathon, Half Marathon and 10K
USATF certified, in 1998 2,000 participants.
Boise, ID
(208) 344-5501 (contact Tim Severa)

Great Southwest Marathon
Abilene, TX
(915) 677-8144

High Plains Marathon
Goodland, KS
(785) 899-5280 (contact Prairie Pacers)

Hogeye Marathon and Relays
USATF certified, in 1998 600 participants.
Fayetteville, AR
(501) 442-6488

Jimmy Stewart Relay Marathon
5 runners split the marathon distance.
Los Angeles, CA
(310) 829-8968
e-mail mbauleke@stjohns.org

Journeys Marathon
USATF certified, in 1998 335 participants.
Eagle River, WI
(800) 359-6315
www.eagleriver.org

Lake County Jenny Spangler Trustmark Marathon
Part of the Lake County Races. USATF certified, in 1998 800 marathon participants, 4,000 participants in all races.
Zion, IL
(847) 266-7223
e-mail Runlakeco@aol.com
www.doitsports.com/lakecountyraces

Lake Geneva Marathon
USATF certified, in 1998 1,000 participants.
Lake Geneva, WI
(414) 248-4323
www.lakegenevasports.com

Lakeland Runaway and Walk on the Wild Side
Vermilion, Alberta, Canada
(403) 853-8474
e-mail margaret.mcmullan@lakelandc.ab.ca

Lincoln Marathon
Lincoln, NE
(402) 435-3504
www.lincolnrun.org

Lone Star Paper Chase Marathon
USATF certified, in 1998 370 participants.
Amarillo, TX
(806) 345-3451
e-mail gnmkt@arn.net

Longest Day Marathon
Brookings, SD
(605) 692-2334
e-mail crober9604@aol.com

Los Angeles Marathon
USATF certified, last year 20,000 participants.
Los Angeles, CA
(310) 444-5544
www.lamarathon.com

Madison Marathon
Madison, WI
(608) 256-9922
www.madison-marathon.com

Maui Marathon and 5K

USATF certified, in 1998 1,300 participants, limited to 1,800.

Kahului, HI

(808) 871-6441

e-mail bark@maui.net

www.mauimarathon.com

Med-City Marathon

Rochester, MN

(507) 282-1411

www.millcomm.com/~adoering/medcity/

Michigan Trail Marathon

In 1998 850 participants.

Ann Arbor, MI

(734) 769-5016(contact Running Fit)

www.apin.com/runfit

Millennium Marathon

Burlington, Ontario, Canada

(905) 639-8053

Muir Woods Marathon

Stinson Beach Park, CA

(415) 868-1829 (contact EnviroSports)

www.envirosports.com

Nantucket Marathon

USATF certified, limited to 500.

Nantucket, MA,

(508) 285-4544

trighost@msn.com

Napa Valley Trail Marathon

Calistoga, CA

(415) 868-1829

www.envirosports.com

National Capital Marathon, Half Marathon, 10K and 5K

USATF certified, in 1998 7,500 participants.

Ottawa, Ontario, Canada

(613) 234-2221

e-mail ncm@storm.ca

www.ncm.ca

New Jersey Shore Marathon

USATF certified, in 1998 1,100 participants.

Long Branch, NJ

(732) 542-6090

e-mail EVART2@aol.com,

www.njshoremarathon.org

Ocean Drive Marathon

Cape May County, NJ

(609) 522-2755

email edepalma@msn.com

Ohio River RRC Marathon, Half Marathon and Relays

USATF certified, in 1998 550 participants.

Xenia, OH

(937) 436-1802

e-mail jsmindak@juno.com

dmiapub.dma.org/orrrc/

Peach City Marathon

Penticton, British Columbia, Canada

(888) 450-3994

e-mail Smbrown@img.net

Pine Line Trail Marathon

Medford, WI

(800) 257-4729

Race of Champions Marathon

Holyoke, MA

(413) 734-0955 (contact Fast Feet)

San Joaquin Valley Marathon, Relays, 5K Run/Walk and 1K Kids' Run

Fresno, CA

(209) 441-1444

e-mail robh@fresnomet.org

Shamrock Sports Fest Marathon, 8K and 5K Walk

USATF certified, in 1998 5,000 participants.

Virginia Beach, VA

(757) 481-5090

e-mail sportsfest@juno.com

Shiprock Marathon, Half Marathon and Relays

USATF certified, in 1998 650 participants.

Farmington, NM

(505) 326-6634

e-mail casa04@sprynet.com

Spring Fling Marathon

Vandalia, OH

(937) 898-7015 (contact Denny Fryman)

Sutter Home Napa Valley Marathon

USATF certified, in 1998 1,800 participants.

Calistoga, CA

(707) 255-2609

e-mail Shnvme@napa.net

www.napa-marathon.com/

Suzuki Rock 'n' Roll Marathon

USATF certified, in 1998 20,000 participants.

San Diego, CA

(619) 450-6510

www.rnrmarathon.com

Trail Breaker Marathon

Waukesha, WI

(414) 453-7600

Trail's End Marathon

Warrenton, OR

(503) 646-7867

www.orrc.net

21st Annual Wild Wild West Marathon, 10-Miler and 3-Miler

USATF certified, in 1998 402 participants.

Lone Pine, CA

(760) 876-4444

e-mail lpcc@gnet.com

Vancouver International Marathon, Half Marathon and 5K Walk

In 1998 6,500 participants.

Stanley Park, Vancouver, British Columbia, Canada

(604) 872-2928

e-mail vim@mindlink.bc.ca

Vermont City Marathon

Burlington, VT

(802) 863-8412

www.vcm.org

Walnut Creek Trail Marathon

Covina, CA

(626) 339-5251 (contact Bill and Cheri Kissell)

Whiskey Row Marathon, Half Marathon, 10K and 2-Mile

In 1998 1,300 participants.

Prescott, AZ

(520) 445-7221 (contact Jen Klement)

Wyoming Marathon and 50-Mile Run

In 1998 75 participants.

Laramie, WY

(307) 635-3316

e-mail RunWyo26point2@compuserve.com

Summer

Big Basin Marathon

Big Basin Redwood State Park, CA

(415) 868-1829 (contact EnviroSports)

www.envirosports.com

Bulldog 50K Ultra Run

Challenging 50K on trails in the Santa Monica Mountains. Send self-addressed stamped envelope for info to:

Ingrid Shattuck

810 Rancho Rd.

Thousand Oaks, CA 91362

(805) 495-2248

Bulldog 30K Run and Hike

Challenging and scenic 30K on trails in the Santa Monica Mountains. Send self-addressed stamped envelope for info to:

Ingrid Shattuck

810 Rancho Rd.

Thousand Oaks, CA 91362

(805) 495-2248

Calgary Stampede Marathon

Calgary, Alberta, Canada

(403) 264-2996

Cambridge Bay Marathon

Cambridge Bay, Northwest Territories, Canada

(212) 288-0786 (contact Tim Decker)

Columbia River Gorge Marathon

Hood River, OR

(503) 697-4787 (contact Lisa Berger)

Crater Lake Rim Marathon

Crater Lake, OR

(541) 884-6939

Des Deux Rives Marathon

Quebec City, Canada

(418) 990-0865

www.marathonquebec.com

Desert News Marathon and 10K

USATF certified, in 1998 4,200 participants.

Salt Lake City, UT

(801) 237-2135

Edmonton Festival Marathon

Edmonton, Alberta, Canada

(403) 433-6062

www.runningroom.com

5th Annual Marathon by the Sea, Half Marathon and 5-Miler

In 1998 500 participants.

St. John, New Brunswick, Canada,

(506) 696-4922

aquatics@nbnet.nb.ca

Fila Sky Marathon and Half Marathon
Aspen, CO
(719) 570-9795
e-mail trlrunner@aol.com

Frank Maier Marathon and Half Marathon
USATF certified, in 1998 110 participants.
Juneau, AK
(907) 586-8322,
e-mail runjuneau@aol.com

Friendly Voyageur Marathon
Massey, Ontario, Canada
(705) 865-2655
massey.etown.net/marathon

God's Country Adelphia Marathon
USATF certified, in 1998 117 participants.
Coudersport, PA
(888) POTTER-2
e-mail potter__county@juno.com

Gold Country Trial Marathon
Nevada City, NV
(530) 878-0697 (contact Nick Vogt)

Grandfather Mountain Marathon
Boone, NC
(828)265-3479 (contact Harry Williams)

Grandma's Marathon
Duluth, MN
(218) 727-0947
www.grandmasmarathon.com

Hoosier Marathon
USATF certified, in 1998 222 participants.
Fort Wayne, IN
(219) 436-2234 (contact Don Lindley)
members.aol.com/vernc3/marathon.htm

Humpy's Classic
Anchorage, AK
(907) 258-4964
www.customcpu.com/np/arc/index.htm

Kilauea Volcano Marathon
Hawaii Volcanoes National Park, Big Island, HI
(808) 735-8733
e-mail jmoberly@lava.net

Kona Marathon, Half Marathon, 10K and 5K
In 1998 450 participants.
Kailua-Kona, HI
(808) 325-0618
e-mail jtl@gte.net

Manitoba Marathon and Half Marathon
Certified course, in 1998 6,800 participants.
Winnipeg, Manitoba, Canada
(204) 925-5751

Marathon de la Baie
Charlo, New Brunswick, Canada
(506) 684-5133

Marathon to Marathon
Storm Lake, IA
(712) 289-2246

Mayo Midnight Marathon
Mayo, Yukon Territory, Canada
(867) 996-2275 (contact Cheryl Klippert)
e-mail mayo@yknet.yk.ca

Mayor's Midnight Sun Marathon
Anchorage, AK
(907) 343-4474
www.ci.anchorage.ak.us

Midnight Sun Marathon
Baffin Island, Northwest Territories, Canada
(867) 436-7502

Mojave 250-Mile Death Race
12-person teams, 21 legs, run and bike, various distances.
NV & CA
(714) 953-4440

Mosquito Marathon
Leadville, CO
(800) 933-3910

Montana Governors Cup Marathon and 20K
USATF certified, in 1998 7,000 participants.
Helena, MT
(800) 447-7828 ext. 3414
www.govcup.bcbsmt.com

Newport Marathon
Newport, OR
(541) 265-3446
www.newportmarathon.org

NipMuck Trail Marathon
In 1998 152 participants.
Ashford, CT
(860) 455-1096

Nova Scotia Marathon
Barrington, Nova Scotia, Canada
(902) 637-2760

Paavo Nurmi Marathon
Upson, WI
(715) 561-4334

Palos Verdes Marathon, Half Marathon and 5K Run/Walk
Palos Verdes, CA
(310) 828-4123 (contact W2 Promotions)
www.w2promo@aol.com

Park City Marathon
Park City, UT
(801) 451-0517
www.pcmarathon.com

Pikes Peak Marathon
In 1998 800 participants.
Manitou Springs, CO
(719) 473-2625

Providian San Francisco Marathon
USATF certified, in 1998 5,000 participants,
San Francisco, CA
(916) 983-4622
e-mail sfm@mgworld.com
www.sfmarathon.com

Rails/Trails Marathon
Brookville, OH
(937) 898-7015 (contact Denny Fryman)

Ridgerunner Marathon
Cairo, WV
(304) 643-2931

Scotty Hanton Marathon, Half Marathon and 8K
USATF certified, in 1998 530 participants.
Port Huron, MI
(810) 987-4932
e-mail dehanton@tir.com

Silver State Marathon
USATF certified, in 1998 1,000 participants.
Reno, NV,
(702) 849-0419
e-mail ski.reno@worldnet.att.net
www.silverstatemarathon.com

South Peace Marathon
Grande Prairie, Alberta, Canada
(780) 532-7138
e-mail turnbl@telusplanet.net

Steamboat Marathon
Steamboat Springs, CO
(970) 879-0880
www.steamboat-chamber.com

Summer Spree Marathon
Vandalia, OH
(937) 898-7015 (contact Denny Fryman)

Sunburst Marathon
South Bend, IN
(219) 674-0090
6262.sunburst.org/

Taos Marathon
Taos, NM
(505) 776-1860
www.emanuelli.com/emad/Marathon-Taos

Tupelo Marathon
Tupelo, MI
(601) 842-2039 (contact Johnny Dye)

2000 Interamerica Millennium Relay Run
From the Canadian Arctic to Tierra del Fuego, South America
(650) 903-0341
e-mail alcatrazjoe@hotmail.com

University of Okoboji Marathon, Half Marathon, 10K and Mini Triathlon
USATF certified, in 1998 425 participants.
Pike's Point State Park, IA
(712) 338-2424

Valley of the Flowers Marathon
Lompoc, CA
(805) 736-3483

Yellowknife Marathon
Yellowknife, Northwest Territories, Canada
(867) 873-2245

Fall

Adirondack Marathon
Schroon, NY
(888) 724-7666
www.adirondackmarathon.org

Aetna U.S. Healthcare Greater Hartford Marathon
USATF certified, in 1998 4,000 participants.
Hartford, CT
(860) 742-7317
e-mail eatnrun@erols.com
www.hartfordmarathon.com

American Odyssey Marathon
Marathon City, WI
(715) 536-1230 (contact Joel Braatz)

Arkansas Marathon
USATF certified, in 1998 160 participants.
Malvern, AR
(501) 337-0007 (contact Dale Burns)

Atlantic City Marathon
Atlantic City, NJ
(609) 601-1786
www.iloveac.com/marathon/

Baton Rouge Beach Marathon
In 1998 189 participants.
Baton Rouge, LA
(504) 275-1576
e-mail brbm@aol.com

Bethel Marathon
Bethel, AK
(907) 543-3213 (contact Mary Krevans)

Bay State Marathon
Tyngsboro, MA
(978) 433-9909
www.baystate.org

Big Island Marathon
Hilo, HI
(800) 984-0506 (contact Wayne Joseph)
e-mail biimara@gte.net

Big Sur Trail Marathon
Carmel, CA
(415) 868-1829
www.envirosports.com

Bismarck Marathon and Half Marathon
USATF certified, in 1998 220 participants.
Bismarck, ND
(701) 255-1525

Burney Classic Marathon
Burney, CA
(530) 335-2825 (contact Don Jacobs)
e-mail dilligas@c-zone.net

Canadian International Marathon
Toronto, Ontario, Canada
(416) 972-1062
www.runtoronto.com

Canadian Rocky Mountain Marathon
Canmore, Alberta, Canada
(403) 678-3332
www.cause.ca/marathon

Cape Cod Marathon
Falmouth, MA
(508) 540-6959
www.capecodmarathon.com

Cynergy Indianapolis Marathon, Half Marathon and 5K
Indianapolis, IN
(317) 826-1670
e-mail joel.sauer@lilly.com

Clarence Demar Marathon
USATF certified.
Gilsum, NH
(877) 526-2379

Detroit Free Press Marathon
USATF certified, in 1998 2,300 participants.
Detroit, MI
(313) 222-7749
www.freep.com

Dutchess County Marathon
Fishkill, NY
(914) 471-0777 (contact Irvin Miller)
www.pojonews.com/dcclassic

Duke City Marathon
Albuquerque, NM
(505) 880-1414
www.dukecitymarathon.com

East Lyme Marathon
USATF certified, in 1998 500 participants.
East Lyme, CT
(860) 739-2864 (contact Way Hedding)

Eriesistible Marathon
USATF certified.
Erie, PA
(814) 456-0621
www.erie.net/~runerie/marathon.htm

Equinox Marathon
Fairbanks, AK
(907) 452-8351 (contact Steve Bainbridge)

Fall Fantasy Marathon
Vandalia, OH
(937) 898-7015 (contact Denny Fryman)

Fox Cities Marathon and Half Marathon
USATF certified, in 1998 2,500 participants.
Menasha, WI
(920) 830-7259
e-mail fcm@execpc.com,
www.runningzone.com/foxcitiesmarathon/

Green Mountain Marathon
South Hero, VT
(802) 434-3228
e-mail hatherton@pipeline.com

Greater Kansas City Marathon
Kansas City, MO
(816) 331-4286
www.kcpl.com

Heart of America Marathon
Columbia, MT
(573) 445-2684 (contact Joe Duncan)

Humboldt Redwoods Marathon and Half Marathon
Weott, CA
(707) 443-1220

Island Marathon, Half Marathon and 10K
In 1998 150 participants.
Charlottetown, Prince Edwards Island
(902) 368-1025
e-mail wlong@city.charlottetown.pe.ca

Johnstown Marathon and 10K
USATF certified, in 1998 225 participants.
Johnstown, PA
(814) 535-8381

KAKE-TV/Wichita Marathon
USATF certified, in 1998 250 participants.
Wichita, KS
(316) 636-1266
www.feist.com/~runwichita

Kokopelli Trail Marathon
Grand Junction, CO
(970) 242-7802
e-mail emgmh@gj.net

Lakefront Marathon
USATF certified.
Milwaukee, WI
(414) 783-5009
e-mail shartman@execpc.com
www.runningzone.com/lakefront

Lake Tahoe Marathon, Run/Walk/Jog, Half Marathon, 10K, 5K and Kids' Fun Run
In 1998 1,625 participants.
Lake Tahoe, CA
(530) 544-7095
e-mail leswright@oakweb.com
www.laketahoemarathon.com

LaSalle Banks Chicago Marathon and 5K
USATF certified, in 1998 20,000 participants.
Chicago, IL
(312) 243-0003
www.chicagomarathon.com

Maine Marathon
Portland, ME
(207) 741-2084
e-mail memarathon@juno.com

Marine Corps Marathon
USATF certified, in 1998 18,300 participants.
Washington, D.C.
(800) RUN-USMC
e-mail marathon@quantico.usmc.mil
www.marinemarathon.com

Mohawk Hudson River Marathon
USATF certified, in 1998 540 participants.
Schenectady, NY
(518) 435-4500
e-mail nypl.albany.net

Montana Marathon
Billings, MT
(406) 248-1685

Mount Rushmore Marathon
Rapid City, SD
(800) 487-3223
www.rapidcitycvb.com

Napa Valley Wine Country Trail Marathon
Calistoga, CA
(415) 868-1829
www.envirosports.com

Newfoundland Provincial Marathon
St. John's, Newfoundland, Canada
(709) 722-9216
www.infonet.st-johns.nf.ca/nfmarathon/

New Hampshire Marathon
Bristol, NH
(603) 744-2649 (contact Fred MacLean)

Niagara Falls Marathon
Niagara Falls, Ontario, Canada
(905) 356-6061
www.tourismniagara.com/nfcvcb

Oilsands Marathon
Fort McMurray, Alberta, Canada
(403) 791-4027 (contact Anne Locke)
e-mail avlp@telusplanet.net

Okanagan Marathon
Kelowna, British Columbia, Canada
(250) 862-3511

Omaha Marathon
Omaha, NE
(402) 398-9807

Portland Marathon, 5-mile Run/Walk and 2-Mile Kids' Run
USATF certified, in 1998 6,000 participants.
Portland, OR
(503) 226-1111
www.portlandmarathon.org

Pueblo River Trail Marathon and Half Marathon
USATF certified, in 1998 400 participants.
Pueblo, CO
(719) 543-5151

Quad Cities Marathon
Moline, IL
(309) 797-1733

The Relay
California's largest party. 12-person team-relay run through 36 cities and across the Golden Gate Bridge, Calistoga to Santa Cruz.
(650) 508-9703
www.therelay.com

Roaring Fork Sunday Marathon
Basalt, CO
(970) 927-9929 (contact John T. Duffy)

Royal Victoria Marathon
Victoria, British Columbia, Canada
(250) 382-8181
www.islandnet.com/~rvm

Sacramento Marathon
USATF certified.
Sacramento, CA
(707) 678-5005
e-mail starlite99@aol.com

St. George Marathon
St. George, UT
(435) 634-5850
www.infowest.com/stgeorgemarathon

St. Louis Marathon
USATF certified, in 1998 800 participants.
St. Louis, MO
(314) 781-3926

Saskatchewan Marathon
Saskatoon, Saskatchewan, Canada
(306) 244-0955

Silicon Valley Marathon
USATF certified, in 1998 5,000 participants.
San Jose, CA
(831) 477-0965
e-mail info@svmarathon.com
www.svmarathon.com

Skagit Flats Marathon
Burlington, WA
(360) 766-6842
e-mail lynnmc@cnw.com

Spokane Series Marathon
Spokane, WA
(509) 624-4297
e-mail joan@gntech.net

Steamtown Marathon
Scranton, PA
(800) 229-3526
www.visitnepa.org

Sugar River Trail Marathon
Brodhead, WI
(608) 862-1596 (contact Sarah Balz)
e-mail sbalz@tds.net

Towpath Marathon
Cleveland, OH
(216) 575-3439

Turtle Marathon
Roswell, NM
(505) 627-5507 (contact Bob Edwards)

Twin Cities Marathon
USATF certified, in 1998 7,500 participants.
St. Paul, MN
(612) 673-0778
www.doitsports.com/marathons/twincities/

United States Air Force Marathon
USATF certified, in 1998 2,500 participants.
Dayton, OH
(800) 467-1823
e-mail thomas.fisher@88abw.wpafb.af.mil

Valley Harvest Marathon
In 1998 400 participants.
Kentville, Nova Scotia, Canada
(902) 542-1867
e-mail moores@glinx.com

Walker North Country Marathon and 10K
USATF certified, in 1998 800 participants.
Walker, MN
(218) 547-3327
e-mail golfisme@paulbunyon.net

Whistlestop Marathon
Ashland, WI
(800) 284-9484
www.ashlandchamber.org/whistlestop

Wineglass Marathon
    Painted Post, NY
    (607) 936-4686
    www.pennynet.org/wineglas

Yonkers Marathon and Half Marathon
    USATF certified, in 1998 340 participants.
    Yonkers, NY
    (914) 377-6430

Ironman Competitions

Blackwater EagleMan Triathlon
    Great Marsh Park, Cambridge, Maryland
    1.2 mile swim • 56 mile bike • 13.1 mile run
    Race Director: Robert Vigorito
    6662 Windsor Court
    Columbia, MD 21044
    Phone: (410) 964-1246
    Fax: (410) 964-2274
    e-mail: rdvigor@erols.com
    www.tricolumbia.org
    Age Group Slots–25

Buffalo Springs Lake Triathlon
    Lubbock, Texas
    1.2 mile swim • 56 mile bike • 13.1 mile run
    Race Directors: Mike and Marti Greer
    P.O. Box 93726
    Lubbock, TX 79493
    Phone: (806) 796-8213
    Fax: (806) 829-2407
    e-mail: greer@windmill.net
    www.greerinc.com
    Wheelchair Division Slots–3 male, 1 female

Half Vineman Triathlon
    1.2 mile swim • 56 mile bike • 13.1 mile run
    P.O. Box 6007
    Santa Rosa, CA 95406
    Phone: (707) 528-1630
    Fax: (707) 523-0577
    e-mail: Vineman@metro.net
    www.vineman.com
    Age Group Slots–25

Ironman Australia Triathlon
    Forster/Tuncurry, N.S.W., Australia
    2.4 mile swim • 112 mile bike • 26.2 mile run
    Race Director: Ken Baggs
    P.O. Box 153, Tuncurry
    N.S.W. 2428, Australia

Phone: (61) (2) 6554-7188
    Fax: (61) (2) 6555-5208
    e-mail: ironman@midcoast.com.au
    www.ironmanoz.com

Ironman Austria Triathlon
    Klagenfurt, Austria
    2.4 mile swim • 112 mile bike • 26.2 mile run
    Race Director: Georg Hochegger
    Domgasse 18
    A-9020 Klagenfurt, Austria
    Phone: (43) 463-509651
    Fax: (43) 463-509 65132 or (43) 463 507 387
    e-mail: Ironman@happynet.at
    www.happynet.at/Ironman

Ironman California Triathlon
    Camp Pendleton, California
    2.4 mile swim • 112 mile bike • 26.2 mile run
    Race Director: Buzz Mills
    P.O. Box 225
    Grimsby, Ontario
    Canada L3M 4G3
    Phone: (905) 945-6216
    Fax: (905) 945-8592
    e-mail: trisport@skylinc.net
    www.ironmancalifornia.com

Ironman Canada Triathlon
    Penticton, British Columbia, Canada
    2.4 mile swim • 112 mile bike • 26.2 mile run
    Codirectors: Chris Gdanski/Barry Poole
    Ironman Canada Race Society
    #104 197 Warren Avenue East
    Penticton, B.C., Canada V2A 8N8
    Phone: (250) 490-8787
    Fax: (250) 490-8788
    e-mail: ironman@vip.net
    For registration information: (905) 945-6216
    www.ironman.ca

Ironman Florida Triathlon

Panama City Beach, Florida
2.4 mile swim • 112 mile bike • 26.2 mile run
Race Director: Jerry Lynch
P.O. Box 225
Grimsby, Ontario
Canada L3M 4G3
Phone: (905) 945-6216
Fax: (905) 945-8592
e-mail: trisport@skylinc.net
www.ironmanflorida.com

Ironman New Zealand Triathlon

Taupo, New Zealand
2.4 mile swim • 112 mile bike • 26.2 mile run
Race Chairman: Paul Gleeson
P.O. Box 74447, Market Road
Auckland, New Zealand
Phone: (64) (9) 522-5346
Fax: (64) (9) 522-5421
e-mail: ironmannz@xtra.co.nz
www.ironman.co.nz

Ironman Pao De Acucar

Porto Seguro, Brazil
2.4 mile swim • 112 mile bike • 26.2 mile run
Race Director: Djan Madruga
Rua Desembargador Paulo Alonson 870
Recreio dos Bandeirantes
Rio De Janeiro-RJ-22790-540
Brazil
Phone/Fax: (55) (21) 490-3642
e-mail: dmadruga@ism.com.br

Ironman Switzerland

Zurich, Switzerland
2.4 mile swim • 112 mile bike • 26.2 mile run
President: Martin Koller
BK Sportpromotion GmbH
Wattstrasse 5, CH-8307 Effretikon
Zurich, Switzerland
Phone: (41) 52 355-1000
Fax: (41) 52 355-1001
e-mail: BKsport@effinet.ch
www.ironman.ch

Ironman USA Lake Placid Triathlon

Lake Placid, New York
2.4 mile swim • 112 mile bike • 26.2 mile run
Race Director: Lyle Harris
P.O. Box 225
Grimsby, Ontario
Canada L3M 4G3
Phone: (905) 945-6216
Fax: (905) 945-8592
e-mail: trisport@skylinc.net
www.ironmanusa.com

Keauhou Kona Triathlon

Kailua-Kona, Hawaii
1.2 mile swim • 56 mile bike • 13.1 mile run
Race Director: Joe Ackles
P.O. Box 2153
Kailua-Kona, HI 96745
Phone: (808) 329-0601
Fax: (808) 326-7329
e-mail: kkt@kona.net
www.ilhawaii.net/kkt
Age Group Slots–25

Lanzarote Ironman Triathlon

Lanzarote, Canary Islands, Spain
2.4 mile swim • 112 mile bike • 26.2 mile run
Race Director: Kenneth Gasque
Club La Santa
35560 Tinajo, Lanzarote
Islas Canarias, Spain
Phone: (34) (928) 59-9995 ext. 4300 or 59-9999
Fax: (34) (928) 59-9993
e-mail: info@ironmanlanzarote.com
www.ironmanlanzarote.com

Quelle Ironman Europe Triathlon

Roth, Germany
2.4 mile swim • 112 mile bike • 26.2 mile run
Race Director: Detlef Kuhnel
Freizeit & Sport Promotion GmbH
Allemannenstrasse 5, D-91174
Spalt, Germany
Phone: (49) 9175-9600 or 9602
Fax: (49) 9175-9601
www.quelle.ironman.de

Index

About the Authors

Mark Allen is the triathlon's Michael Jordan. He is a six-time winner of the Ironman Triathlon held in Hawaii (his final victory came at the age of thirty-seven, making him the event's oldest champion ever), a ten-time undefeated champion of the Nice International Triathlon, the sport's only triple crown winner (he won the Ironman Triathlon, the Nice Triathlon, and the demanding Zofingen duathlon all in one year), and the only triathlete in history to have a twenty-race winning streak. **Julie Moss**, an internationally known triathlete, is a three-time Japan Ironman champion and Masters marathoner. Mark and Julie live in Northern California with their son, Mats. **Bob Babbitt** is the cofounder and editor of Competitor Publishing, which publishes *Competitor Magazine*, *CitySports Magazine*, and *Florida Sports Magazine*, among others. He lives in Southern California.